We dedic

Grady, Maura & Conor
~
Our mother passed away from breast cancer

Miranda
~
My father has pancreatic cancer

Hayden
~
My father passed away from melanoma

Justin
~
My mother is a lymphoma survivor

Jennifer
~
My father passed away from a brain tumor

Zack
~
My mother has breast cancer

Cole
~
My mother is a thyroid cancer survivor

Christina
~
My mother is an ovarian cancer survivor

Sarah
~
My father passed away from pancreatic cancer

Lydia
~
My mother has breast cancer

Michael
~
My mother has pancreatic cancer

Brendan
~
My mother passed away from lung cancer

Jennifer
~
My father passed away from brain cancer

Kelly
~
My mother passed away from a brain tumor

Devon
~
My mother has breast cancer

Nick
~
My mother passed away from breast cancer

Allison & Erika
~
Our father passed away from lung cancer

Wynne
~
My mother passed away from breast cancer

Wesley
~
My father is a lymphoma survivor

Sarah
~
My father is a brain tumor survivor

A THANK YOU TO ALL WHO MADE THIS BOOK POSSIBLE...

The Teens

Devon
Cole
Michael
Brendan
Wesley
Allison & Erika
Christina
Kelly
Jennifer
Hayden
Wynne
Zack
Nick
Miranda
Grady, Maura & Conor
Justin
Sarah
Jennifer
Lydia

The Crew

Andrew Mitchell, illustrations
Cheryl Dow, legal
Courtney Herrmann, editing
Dave Peters, Kids Konnected
Debra Nelson, graphic design
Elizabeth Borsting, publicity
Lynnette Wilhardt LCSW, Shrink Wrap Doc
Sarah Nance, art director / graphic design

A donation of $5 will be made to Kids Konnected from the sale of every book to support their mission and teens like you.

ISBN 0-9768605-4-6
Published by Recipe For Success Incorporated

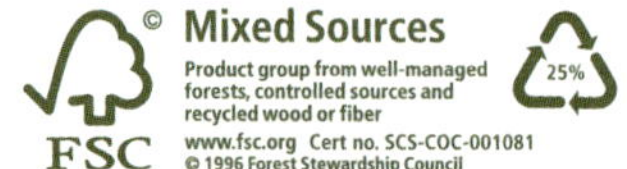

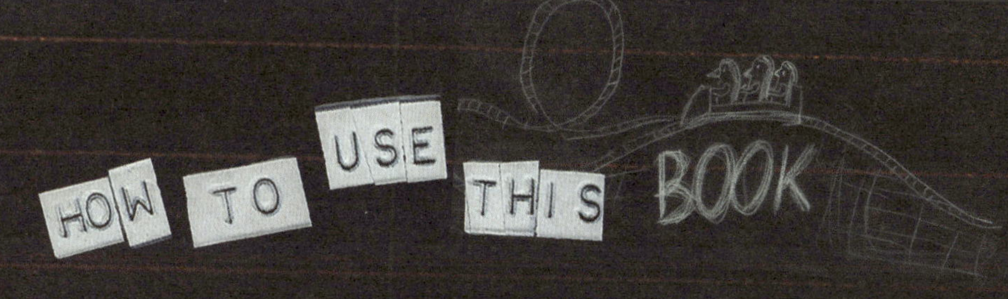

The first book I used in a group setting had a yellow spiral binding and penguins drawn on it. Not artistic penguins, whatever that means. They wore scarves and rode around on roller coasters, they were black, white, yellow and lime green. The pages were filled with questions: How do you feel after school? What planet would you send cancer too? I was fourteen at the time, so I answered the questions dutifully amidst the penguins.

I mean, after all, they were good questions. How did I feel after school? (Glad to be home.) And what planet would I send cancer too? (Mars, I guess, it's really hot right?) But although the penguins were cute, they didn't have a voice to share with me. The page was blank except for my thoughts, and the colors didn't expand off the page. My feelings however, my emotions, my anger, all that stuff I had dealt with, especially after my mom died, went beyond page expansion. They filled my brain like a full balloon, helium threatening to explode my skull. When it couldn't escape from my head, it settled like a lion satisfied with a small steak, into my chest where it angrily reminded me of its presence whenever life seemed to get normal.

I could've used a voice from those penguins, to tell me they knew how I felt, or that they had no idea how I felt but they too, hated cancer and what it had done to their lives. I have always been fairly good at expressing my feelings, but it always seemed that my raw ability to say it how it is made others afraid of how to respond. What could they say back to me about my mom? Could they ask me how I was? Could they talk about how they had just gone with their mom to the mall when I hadn't done that in forever? My friends were at a loss of how to remember my mom themselves, and how to approach the way I was feeling. Damn those silent penguins.

Consider us, the artists, poets, writers, bloggers, creative makers. You are not alone. We have emotions that are not hidden amongst these pages. They are real, they are honest, they are ours. But they are yours too. All of us who have had parents with cancer share these emotions at some point, and some of us are good at expressing them and others aren't. When you come to this book, view it as an open door, an invitation. If you have a story to share, scrawl it on the book pages themselves, or take the idea to a notebook. If an image resounds in your head, draw it, paint it, take a photo of it. This book is full of voices that want you to hear their story, and inspire you to share your own.

We welcome you to contribute your story. You are not alone.

Wynne
March 2008

Throughout this book we've included SHRINK wrap pages to help you understand the "why" behind different actions and feelings you may be experiencing.

*These pages were written by Lynnette, a therapist who specializes in working with families who have a parent with cancer... so you could think of it as **customized** therapeutic advice.*

Take from them what you will, and hopefully there's something you come across that CLICKS with you.

Having a little insight never hurt,
and who knows....
it might be a helpful guide in making
good decisions for yourself.

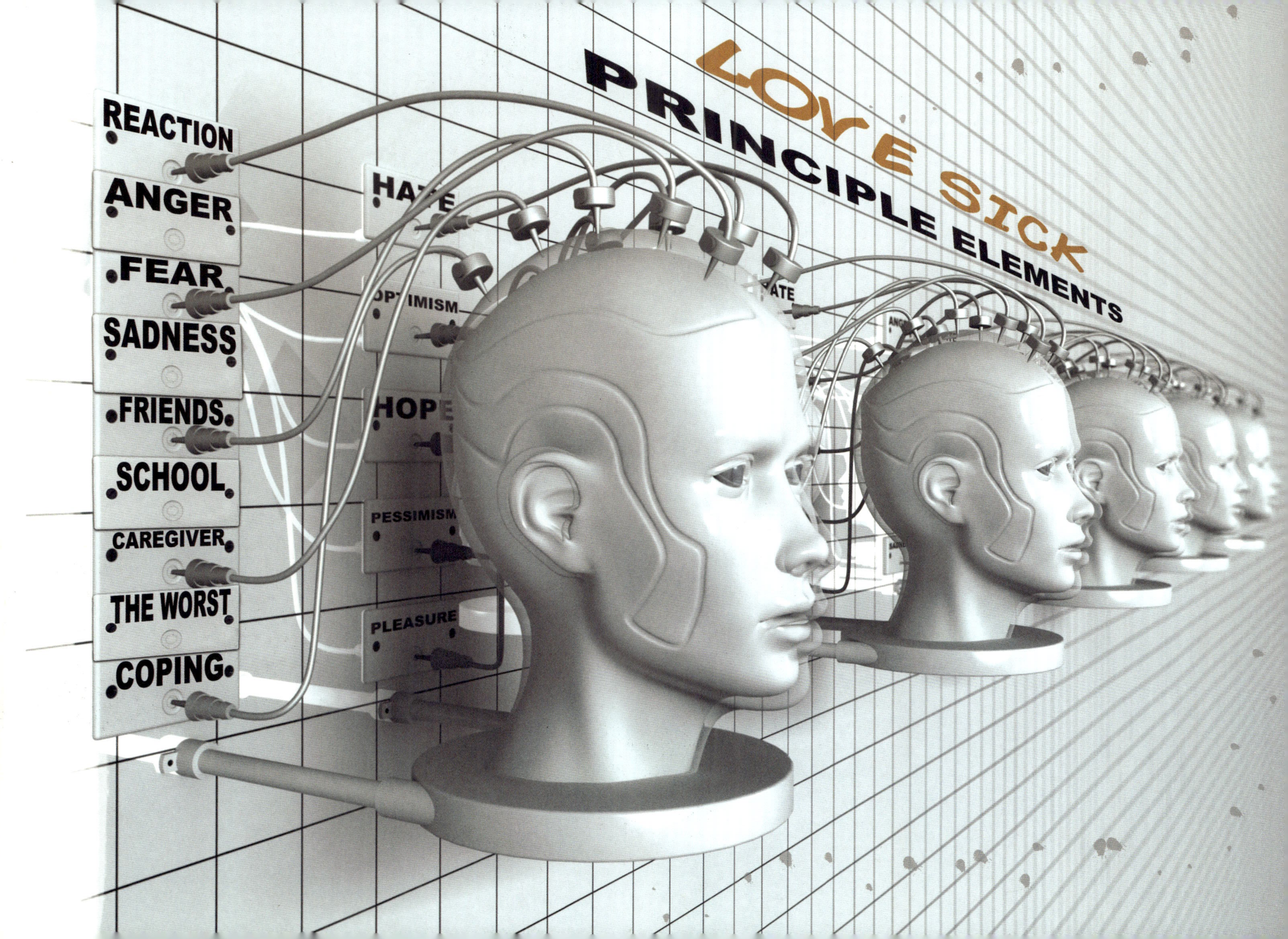
LOVE SICK
PRINCIPLE ELEMENTS
REACTION
ANGER
FEAR
SADNESS
FRIENDS
SCHOOL
CAREGIVER
THE WORST
COPING
OPTIMISM
HOPE
PESSIMISM
PLEASURE

Some days are ingrained in your mind forever;

some are boring,

some are exciting,

AND SOME CHANGE YOUR LIFE.

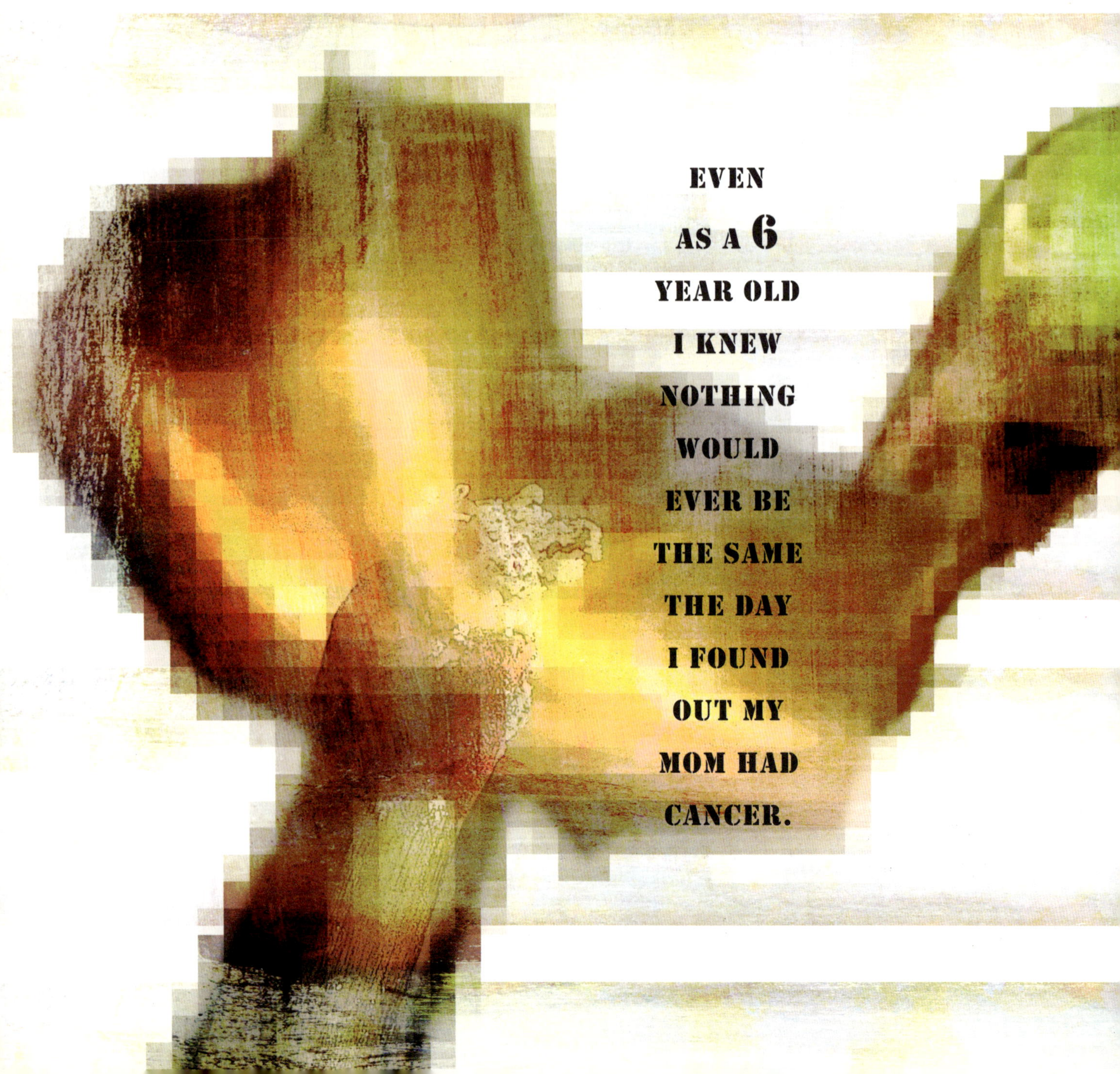

When I woke up that morning, I didn't think, today mom is going to end up in the hospital. It started out as any other morning, my dad went to work, my mom dropped me off at school, dropped my sister at preschool and then she went to work at the elementary school where she taught third grade. **During a meeting at the school district office, my mom had a seizure.** Her co-workers called 911 and she was rushed to the hospital. It didn't take long to identify the cause of the seizure, and she immediately underwent emergency brain surgery to remove the tumor. She was in the hospital for about a week recovering and trying to figure out where to get the best treatment.

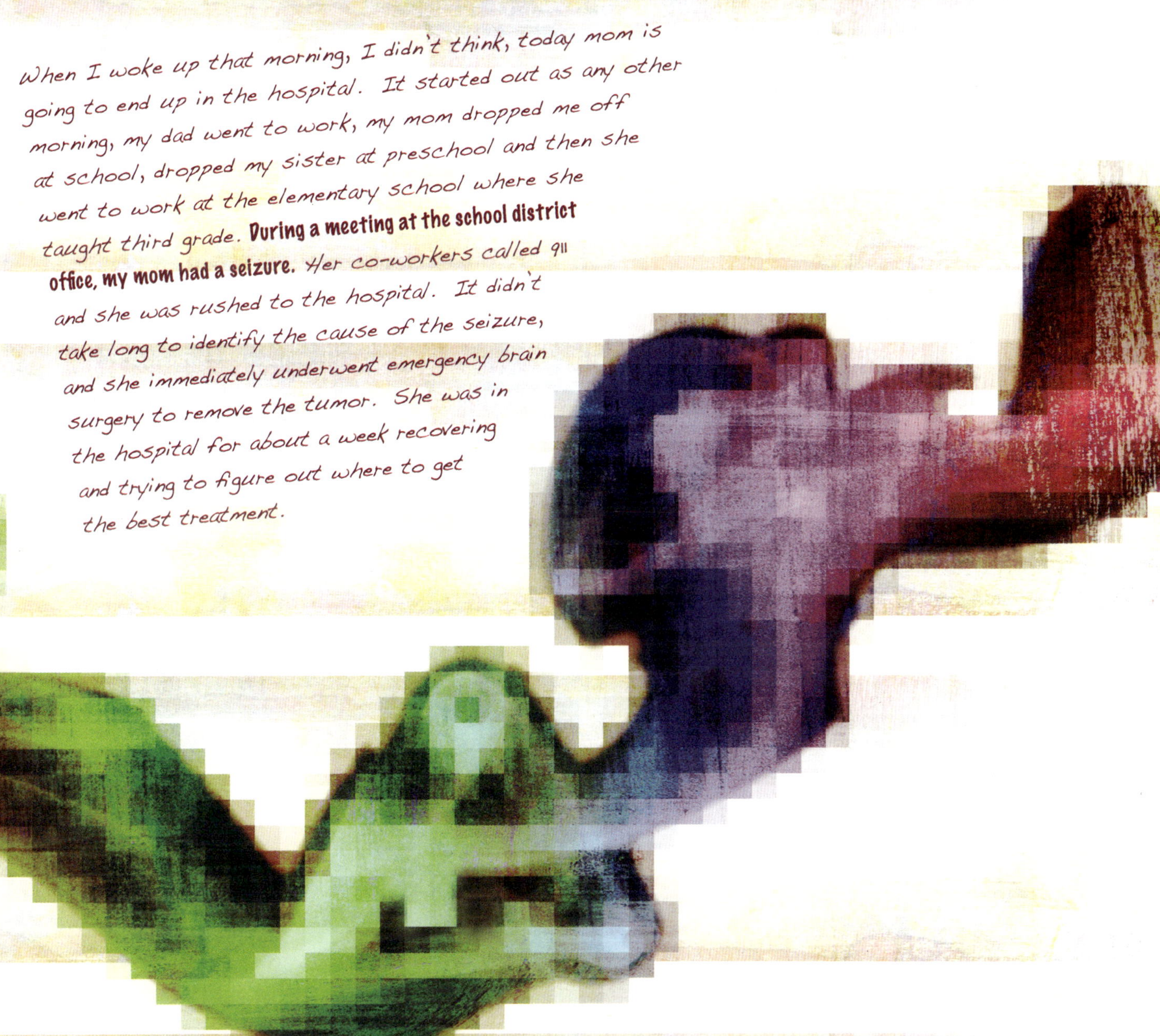

Cancer is such a foreign word to a young child and I think I was too young to completely grasp the complete meaning of the diagnosis. I was still a little girl in first grade, so some of my exact memories of the day and of that week have become fuzzy, but with the help of family I have been able to sort out how I was affected that day. There are many other days have shaped who I have become and defined the obstacles that I have had to overcome. But the day my mom was diagnosed with brain cancer was the first of them all.

– Kelly

A MAN HAS NO MORE CHARACTER THAN HE CAN COMMAND IN A TIME OF CRISIS.

ANONYMOUS

HOPE

guilt process remember failure ANGER scared PRETEND frustration numb love tears pain fear inside PROTECT emotion reaction community terrified STRUGGLE d-i-s-c-o-n-n-e-c-t-e-d express ANXIOUS embarrassed understand difficult Lonely unfair

memories friendship faith courage support feelings ESCAPE difficult OBLIGATION avoid denial CONFLICT

REALITY

by Wesley

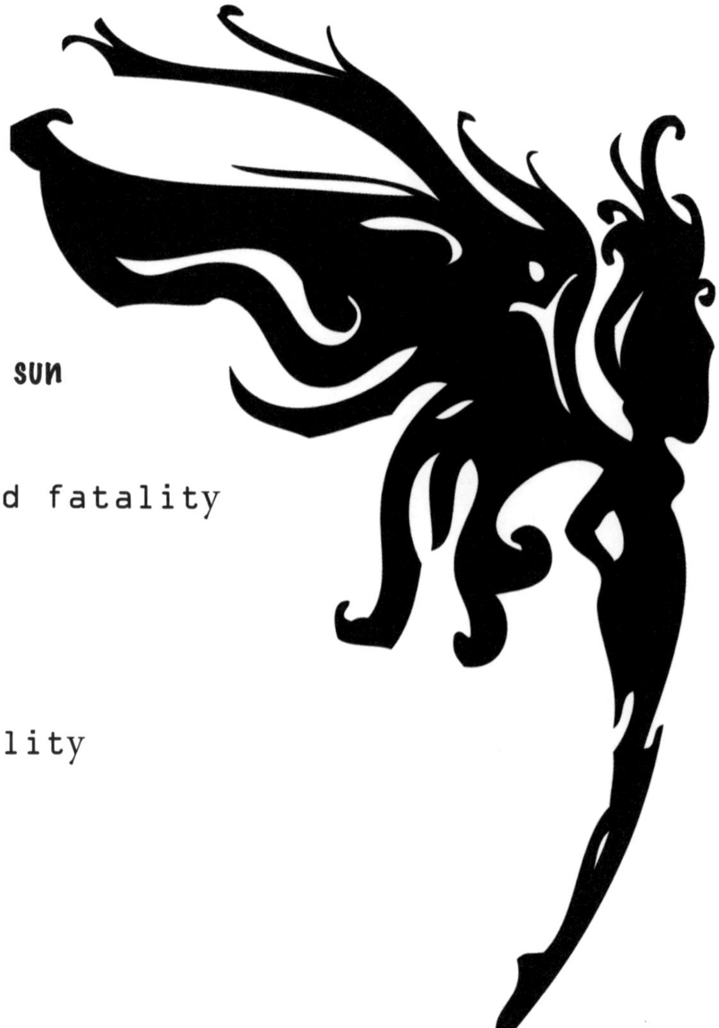

Kept in the **dark**ness of the **sun**

Deluded **visions** of worship and fatality

The outdone soon **undone**

Abolished lie **the lines** of reality

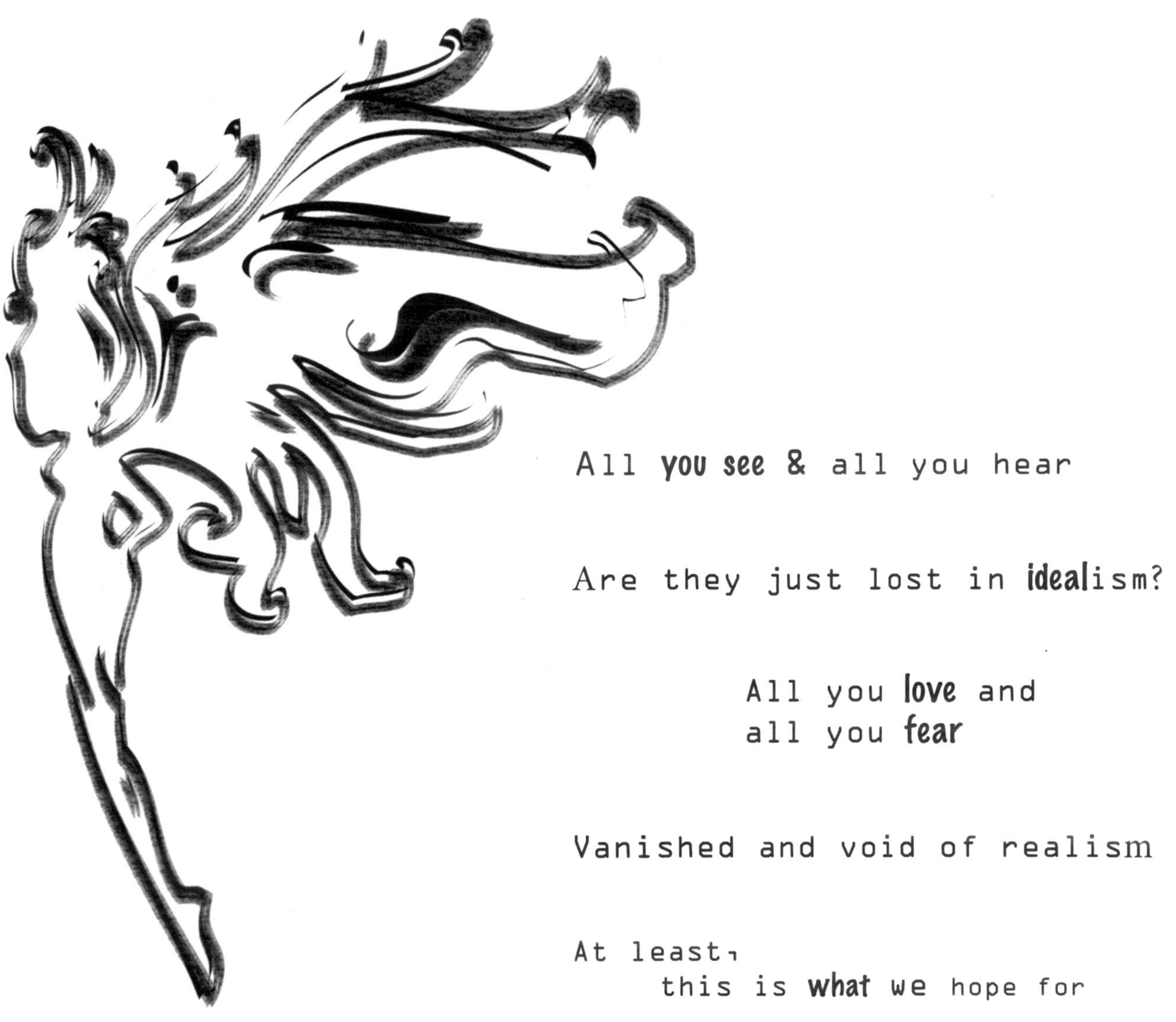

All **you see** & all you hear

Are they just lost in **ideal**ism?

All you **love** and
all you **fear**

Vanished and void of realism

At least,
this is **what** we hope for

i forgive your body

by wynne

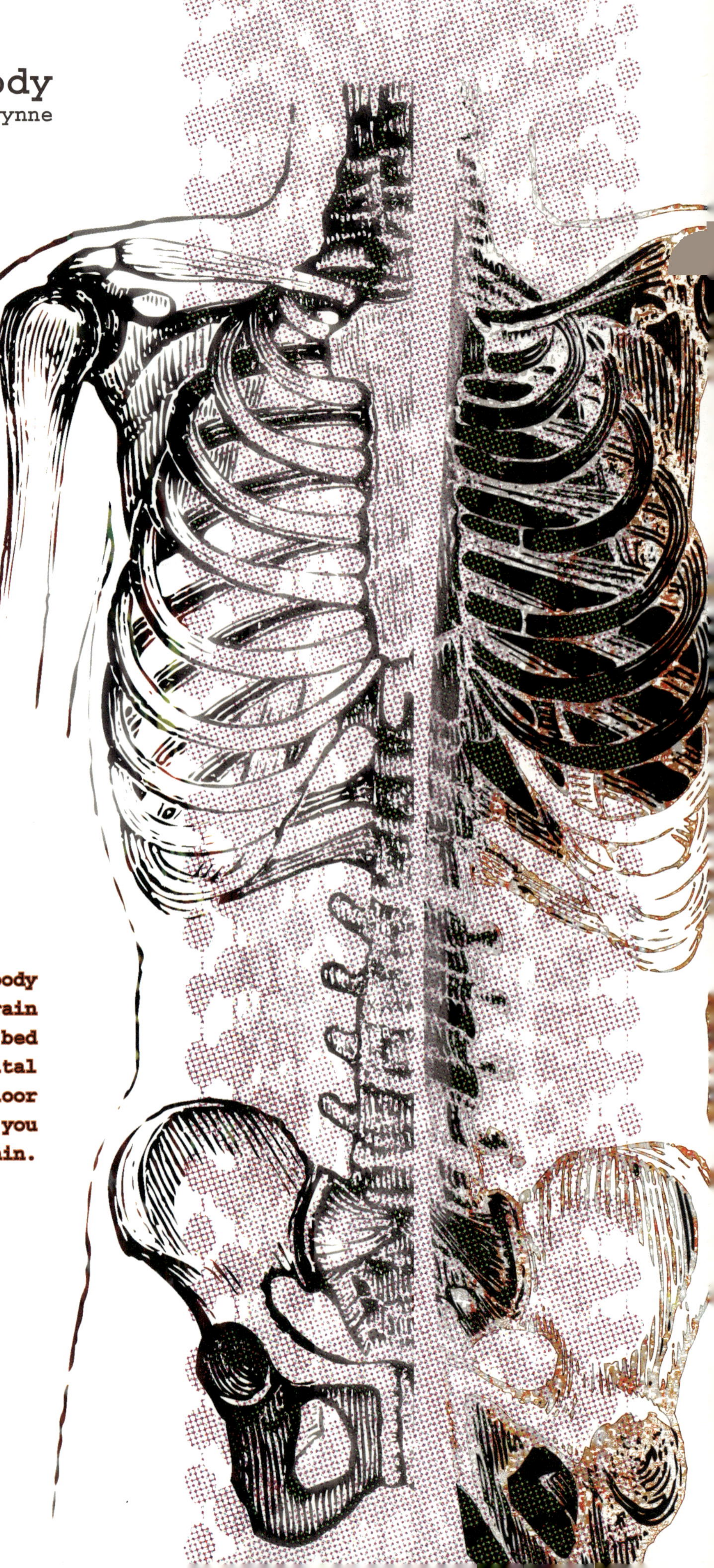

i forgive your body
skin the color of olives
eyelids like moss
thing today, too long legs
i forgive your body for its
loss.

i forgive your body
for exposing your spine
wet, bloody skin as you bent
over
for me to bandage the bone
i forgive your body for
running short on time.

i forgive your body
when your kidneys quit
liters of fluid filling you
like a full womb
i forgive your body for its spit.

i forgive your body
letting go before your brain
you had a job, it kept you in bed
a child, not the hospital
syringes covering the bathroom floor
i forgive your body for causing you
pain.

i forgive your body
for setting you free
as your eyes look into the lense
I see how desperately you fought
how deeply you needed freedom
and yet still.

i cannot forgive your body
for what it did to me.

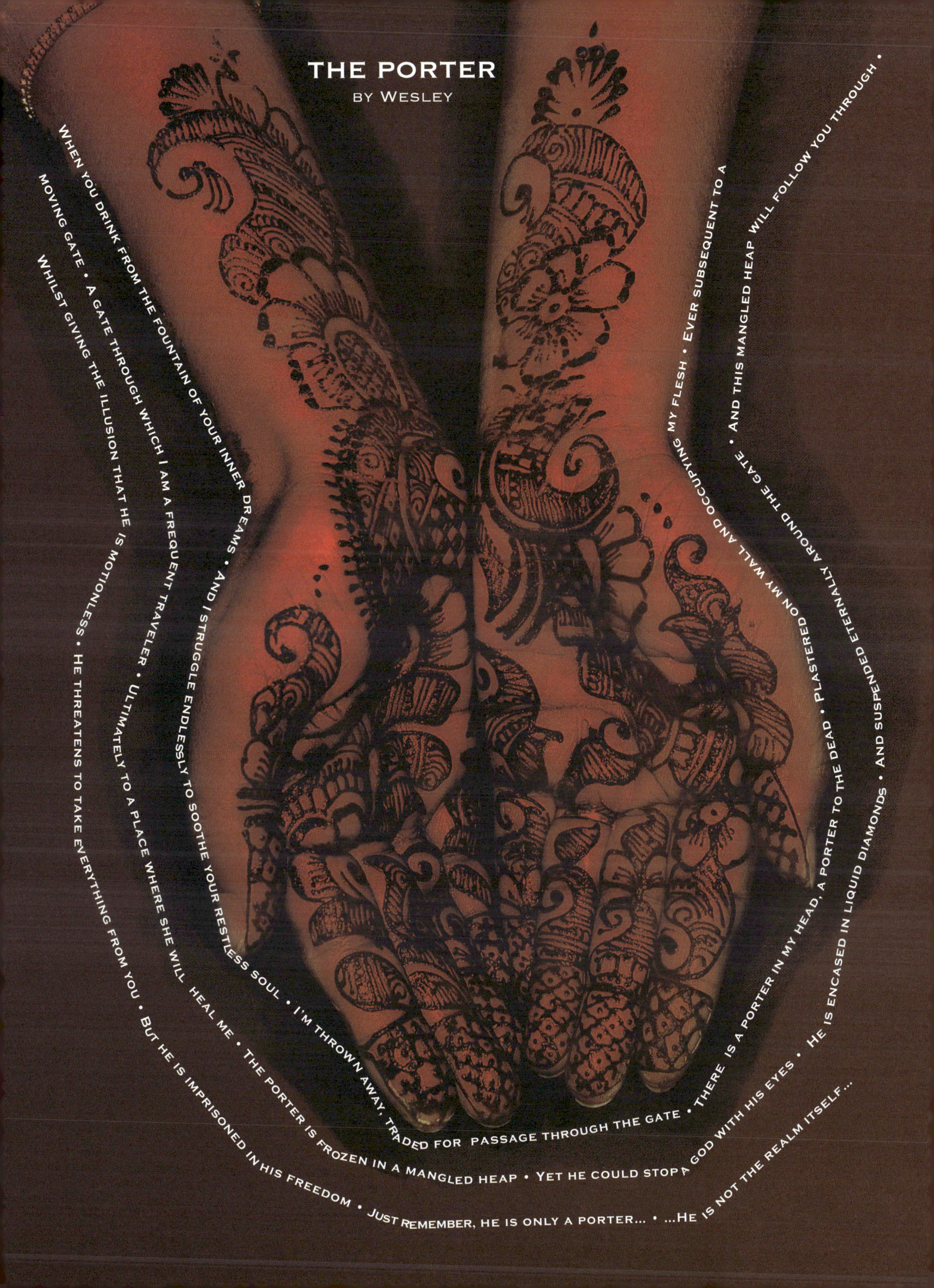

The Porter

By Wesley

When you drink from the fountain of your inner dreams • And I struggle endlessly to soothe your restless soul • I'm thrown away, traded for passage through the gate • There is a porter in my head, a porter to the dead • Plastered on my wall and occupying my flesh • Ever subsequent to a moving gate • A gate through which I am a frequent traveler • Ultimately to a place where she will heal me • The porter is frozen in a mangled heap • Yet he could stop a god with his eyes • He is encased in liquid diamonds • And suspended eternally around the gate • And this mangled heap will follow you through • Whilst giving the illusion that he is motionless • He threatens to take everything from you • But he is imprisoned in his freedom • Just remember, he is only a porter... • ...He is not the realm itself...

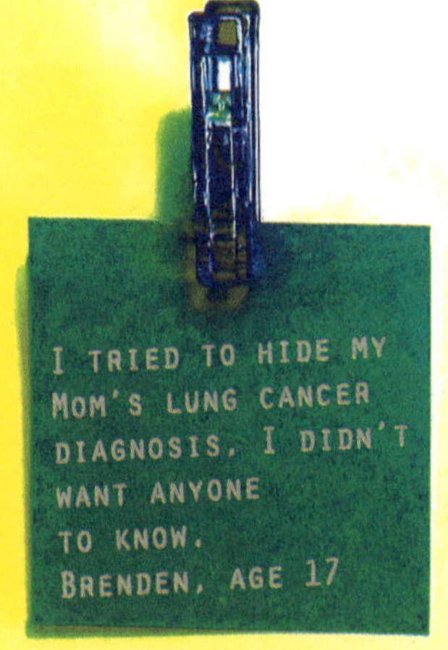

I DIDN'T HAVE A VERY BIG REACTION UNTIL CHEMOTHERAPY. ONCE DAD DID HAVE CHEMO AND LOST HIS HAIR, I BEGAN TO REALIZE THE SEVERITY OF THINGS.
WESLEY, AGE 16

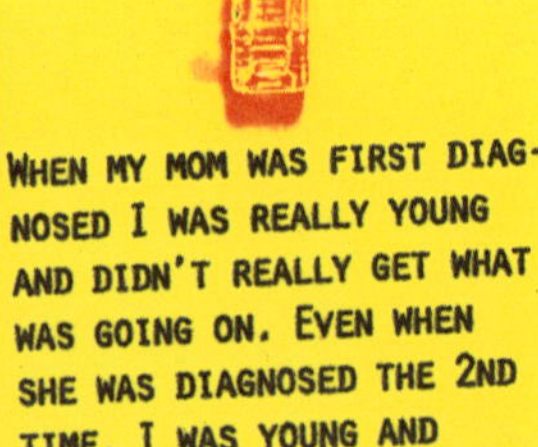

BY THE 3RD RECURRENCE, I HAD A DRAMATIC REACTION. I'M VERY CLOSE TO MY MOM AND SEEING THE EFFECTS OF CHEMO MADE IT REAL AND BEING OLDER MADE ME BETTER ABLE TO UNDERSTAND. I WAS SCARED. ZACK, AGE 15

What your reaction may feel like

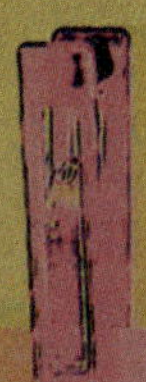

When my Mom was diagnosed with ovarian cancer I was only 9 years old. I was embarrassed when she lost her hair. Now as a teen, I feel bad I was so embarrassed, I didn't know how sick she was, how close to death. I'm grateful she is still alive. Christina, age 15

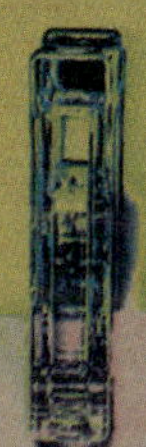

I didn't really have any particular reaction when my mom was diagnosed with pancreatic cancer. It kind of didn't hit me right away. I just remember her having it, I don't remember being told. Since →

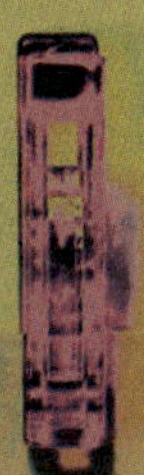

it is only my mom and I at home, I hide my feelings, but have also fully accepted it and am ready to move on. I vent with skateboarding. Michael, age 15

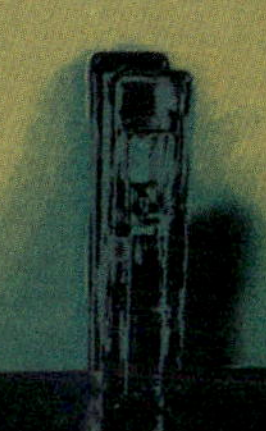

I cried a lot when my mom told me she had breast cancer. I was really young, but I think I would still react the same way. Devon, age 16

It's like hitting a brick wall It's like falling and hitting bottom

It's like running as fast as you can and tripping over a root that wasn't there a second ago

And it's like not feeling anything at all

You're listening to the word, you're hearing the words, but something inside you is saying that this is something big, something awful and it's going to change the rest of your life. Your parent is telling you that they have lymphoma, they have breast cancer, they have leukemia, they have lung cancer, they have multiple myeloma, they have a brain tumor. What are they talking about? At this point you're not even listening any more, it feels too hazy, too soft to be reality is this really happening to me? When am I going to wake up?

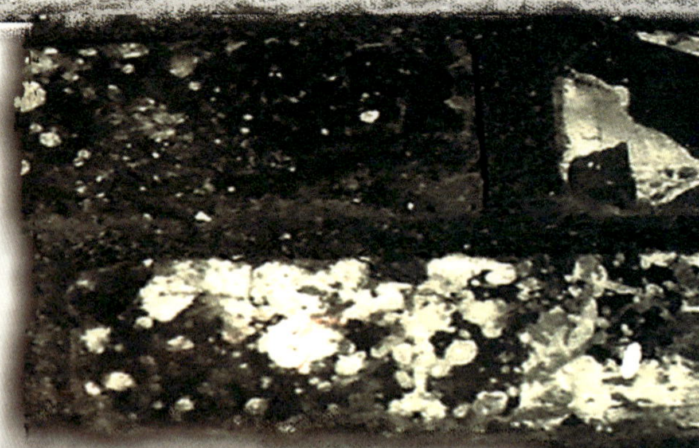

At first you might feel numb.
Try to pretend you really didn't just hear that your parent has cancer. You might just try to get on with your life as you normally do, and salvage the situation.

Maybe you get on with your life a little faster.

Maybe you stay out of the house more, avoid the family more, just avoid the entire situation in an attempt to try to put it behind you. But this isn't something you can put behind you, because when you walk back in the door, it's still there. It's hard enough to be a teen. Just trying to fit in, keep friends, stay out of trouble, get good grades, get into a good college. I mean the pressure can be overwhelming at times. But add to it a parent getting cancer or even worse, dying….well, that's just the final straw.

I know, however, that my story is not unique and that there are thousands of us going through the same experience, the same feelings and the same frustrations. I wrote this book with many others because there isn't any book out there written for teens, by teens and I just didn't think adults really "got" what we are going through.

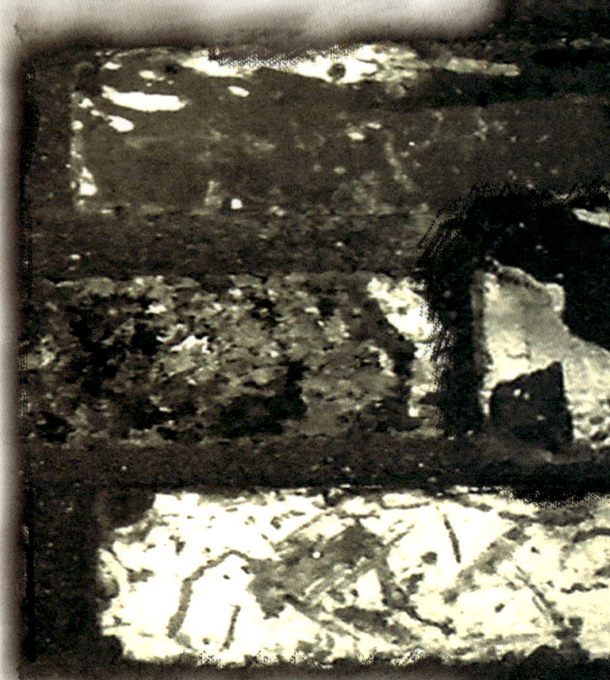

I hope that this book helps you understand the journey you are on or going to be on.

I hope it helps a little with all the feelings you will be experiencing and I hope it helps you feel a little less crazy and a little less lonely out there.

Grady, 17 years old

It is always difficult to face a parent's illness, but it can be even more challenging for a teen.

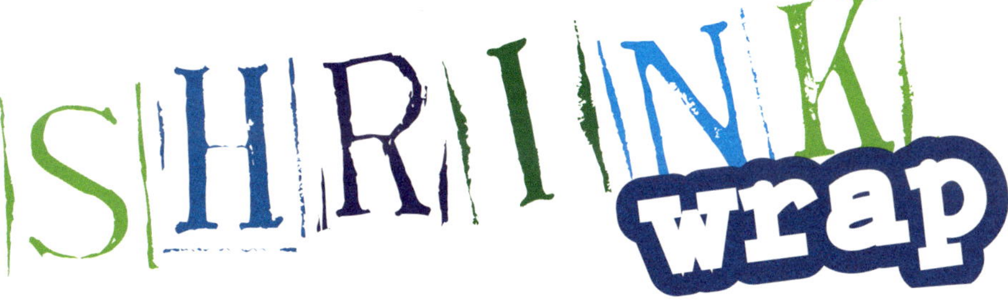

As you approach this time of individuation, your natural inclination will be to move away from your parents. **When a parent is diagnosed with cancer this individuation process becomes complicated.** You may struggle between wanting to leave and be with your friends and feeling a sense of guilt and obligation to remain close to your sick parent. You may not even realize this conflict is going on and instead may find yourself staying increasingly away from home and in complete denial that you are trying to avoid the stressors of home life.

As a teen, you are not quite accessing all the parts of your brain yet. Most teens function primarily with their ***amygdale***. That is the emotional center of your brain. This is the part of the brain that is responsible for all the impulsiveness in your actions and all the emotional drama that goes on in high school. You won't be accessing the frontal lobe of your brain until early adulthood. THE FRONTAL LOBE IS THE PART OF THE BRAIN THAT HELPS WITH ORGANIZED AND RATIONAL THINKING. So, trust me, this is not a time of your life when you will be making your best decisions.

So, it just might make sense to smoke a little pot every day to take the edge off of all the stress you are feeling. The problem with this thinking is that the pot habit will eventually lead to more depression, more irritability and more anxiety, which really only multiplies your problems. It doesn't take anything away.

Adolescence is also an egocentric age and it may be difficult to see beyond yourself long enough to realize the "need" a parent might have for you to be at home. While in this "escape mode", many teens can get into trouble as they try to cope with their feelings regarding their parent's illness. Some will try to escape and numb their feelings with drugs and alcohol. Others will try to externalize their feelings and pain through self mutilation. Others will try to "control" certain aspects of their life which can manifest itself in an eating disorder or school phobia.

Hopefully with some insight, support and therapeutic help, you can avoid more serious problems and deal with this unfair adversity in you life in a healthy, positive way.

- Lynnette

ANGER

When the anesthesia wears off and you are no longer numb you might start to feel anger. Instead of numb, you start to let the feelings rush to your head. By the time the angry rush of adrenaline hits you, you're already feeling better. Anger is a power trip. Being angry has made you feel powerful and in control. Anger makes the problem feel like it's nothing you can't handle. The kick is that you need something to focus your anger on. Family, friends, complete strangers and even yourself may become the victim of this anger. It has made you feel better, but it has also hurt those around you. Anger is a quick fix, one that helps your current state of mind, numbing the consequences of your actions and alienating yourself from others. The only thing left for anyone else is a cold angry person in your place. Now this cold angry person can be pretty tough to get along with. You might find yourself fighting a lot with your siblings, friends or parents. These are not your best outlets, but they may be impossible to avoid. Other outlets may be music, sports or friends. Diversion can be helpful to get your mind off the seriousness and pain you may be going through.

Grady, 18

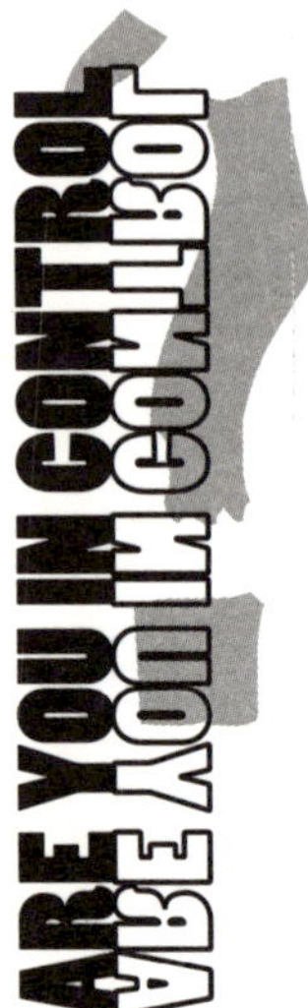

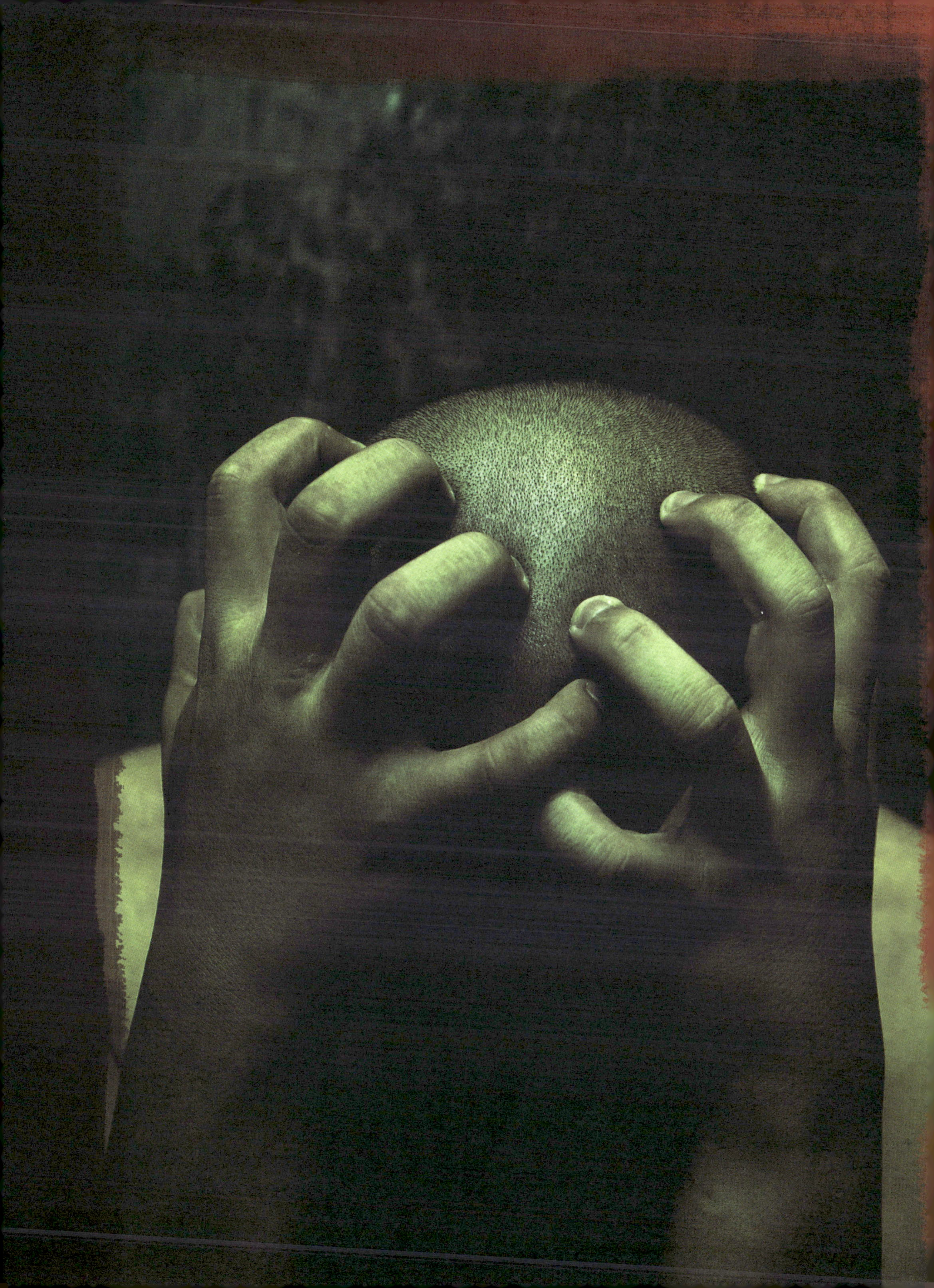

PAGES have been left intentionally
blank throughout the book

USE them to draw, to write or whatever

make this book your own

my anger FEELS LIKE
a release of pain
AND let go FROM THE build-up
of emotions

my anger is me hiding
behind the PAIN I've
experienced IN the past

MY ANGER is
A result OF THE PAIN
i've experienced

MY ANGER IS USEFUL because it
helps me express the frustration THAT LIES
WITHIN ME other than that. it's not useful.
there ARE other WAYS that i could express
myself other than by being AN ANGRY PERSON

Jess 16

NEWS UPDATE

by wynne

Mom.
i've done well for the most part
walked straight
made good use of my heart
as i make the move to school
my feelings lump
my excitement pools.

Mom.
my veins and tendons
muscles spill
all over and although
a mess-
still
i am angry at you
i could be rejoicing instead
it's true- everything i do
ruined.

Mom.
i need a pair of high heels
to crush all of what i feel
how you left, not nice
not quiet and not polite
in the grand scheme of things
the worst thing you did right.

Mom.
i've been the victim since the
fourteenth
and if truth be told
been getting by
by the skin of my teeth
asking for favors that don't
receive
damn these teeth.

Mom.
every event that passes by
in each second of my Get By Life
is covered in the part of you that
stayed
i mourned those pieces for awhile
you know- your laugh, our smile
those really just got in my way.

Mom.
i'm tired of feeling sad
i'm exhausted of everything else
i'm mad
i'm mad at you for your life
why did you have to be my only friend
i'm mad at The End.

I know I'm acting **angry**. . .

but **I'm** really feeling sad

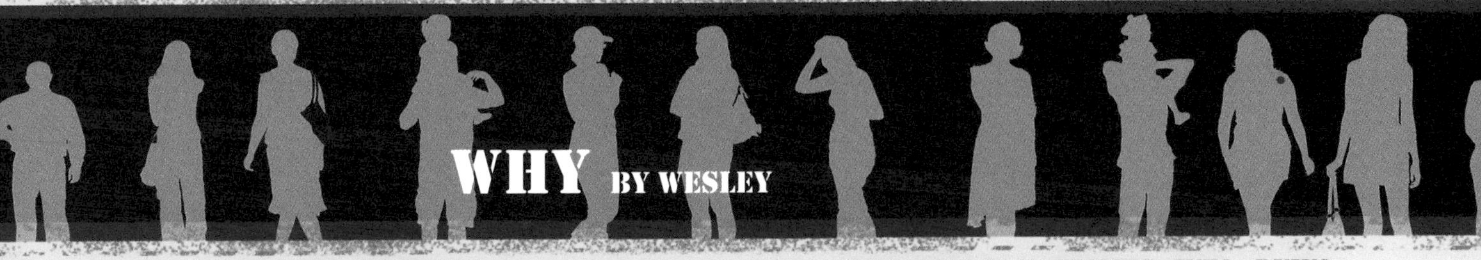

WHY BY WESLEY

WHY ARE YOU?
WHY DO WE NEED YOU?
WHY DO WE BOTHER WITH YOU?
WHY DO WE HOLD ON TO YOU?
WHY CAN'T WE SEE YOU
ONLY DESTROY US?

WHY ARE YOU FALLING INTO RUIN?
WHY ARE YOU TAKING OTHERS WITH YOU?
WHY DID YOU LET THIS HAPPEN TO
YOURSELF?
WHY DIDN'T SOMEONE NOTICE THIS?
WHY DOES CHANGE REQUIRE REVOLUTION?

WHY CAN'T WE LET YOU GO?
WHY SHOULD I FOLLOW YOU?
WHY SHOULD I OBEY?
WHY SHOULD I CONFORM TO YOU?
WHY SHOULD I STAY HERE?
WHY SHOULD I BE?
WHY SHOULD I DO AS YOU DO?

WHY DOES CHANGE REQUIRE DEATH?
WHY MUST WE UNIFY OUR BELIEFS?
WHY MUST WE DESTROY
WHAT'S "UNACCEPTABLE?"
WHY GOVERNMENT?
WHY ECONOMY?
WHY RELIGION?
WHY UNIFICATION?

WHY SHOULD I HAVE YOUR VALUES?
WHY SHOULD I HATE YOU?
WHY SHOULD I LOVE YOU?
WHY ARE YOU BLEEDING?
WHY ARE YOU DOING THIS
TO YOURSELF?

WHY OVER-POPULATION?
WHY CRUELTY TO ANIMALS?
WHY CRUELTY TO HUMANS?
WHY CRUELTY TO PLANETS?
WHY CAPITALISM?
WHY OVER-STIMULATION?
WHY THIS SOCIETY?

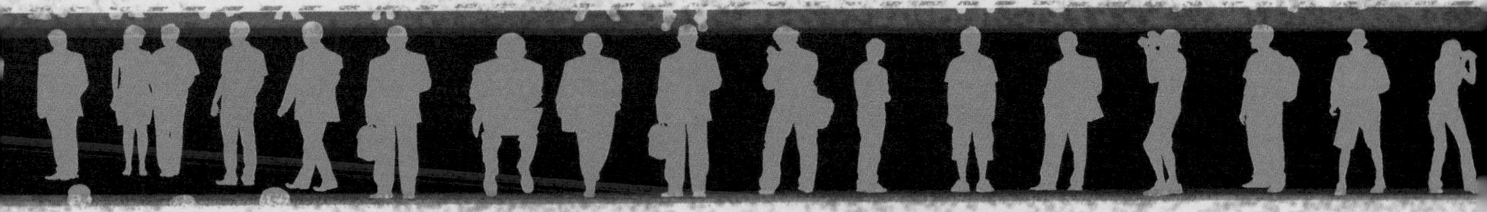

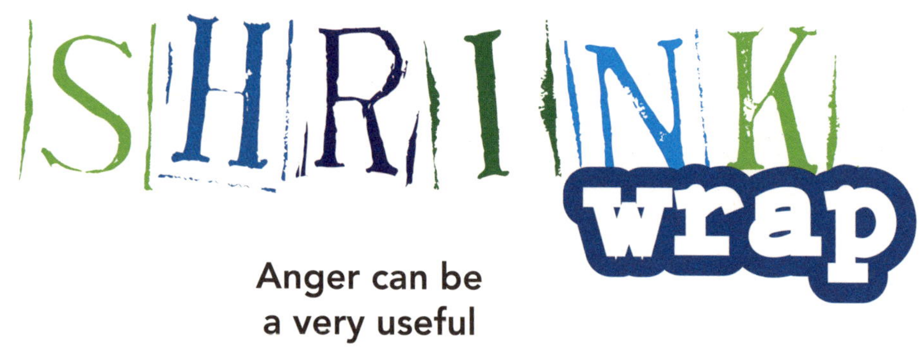

Anger can be a very useful emotion.

It helps us protect ourselves and lets people know that they have done something that upsets us. We use our anger to try to make a change. The problem with anger is that sometimes we become gluttons with it and hoard it inside of ourselves, in an attempt to protect ourselves. When you store too much of it inside of yourself, it becomes your only accessible emotion. So you take out your anger when you're sad, or frustrated or lonely or anxious.

Anger becomes a habit and the natural reaction to everything becomes anger. And then you become an "angry person." Anger isn't meant to be stored inside of ourselves. You have to think of anger like the "hot potato game." You want to get rid of it as soon as you can.

Get your anger out, express your feelings to whomever you are angry with, then let it go. ***Don't harbor the anger inside of you, as it will only grow and fester inside of you.*** Other ways to deal with anger are to exercise, listen to music, or talk to someone you trust.

- Lynnette

Bad habits are like
a comfortable bed,
easy to get into,
but hard to get out of.

Anonymous

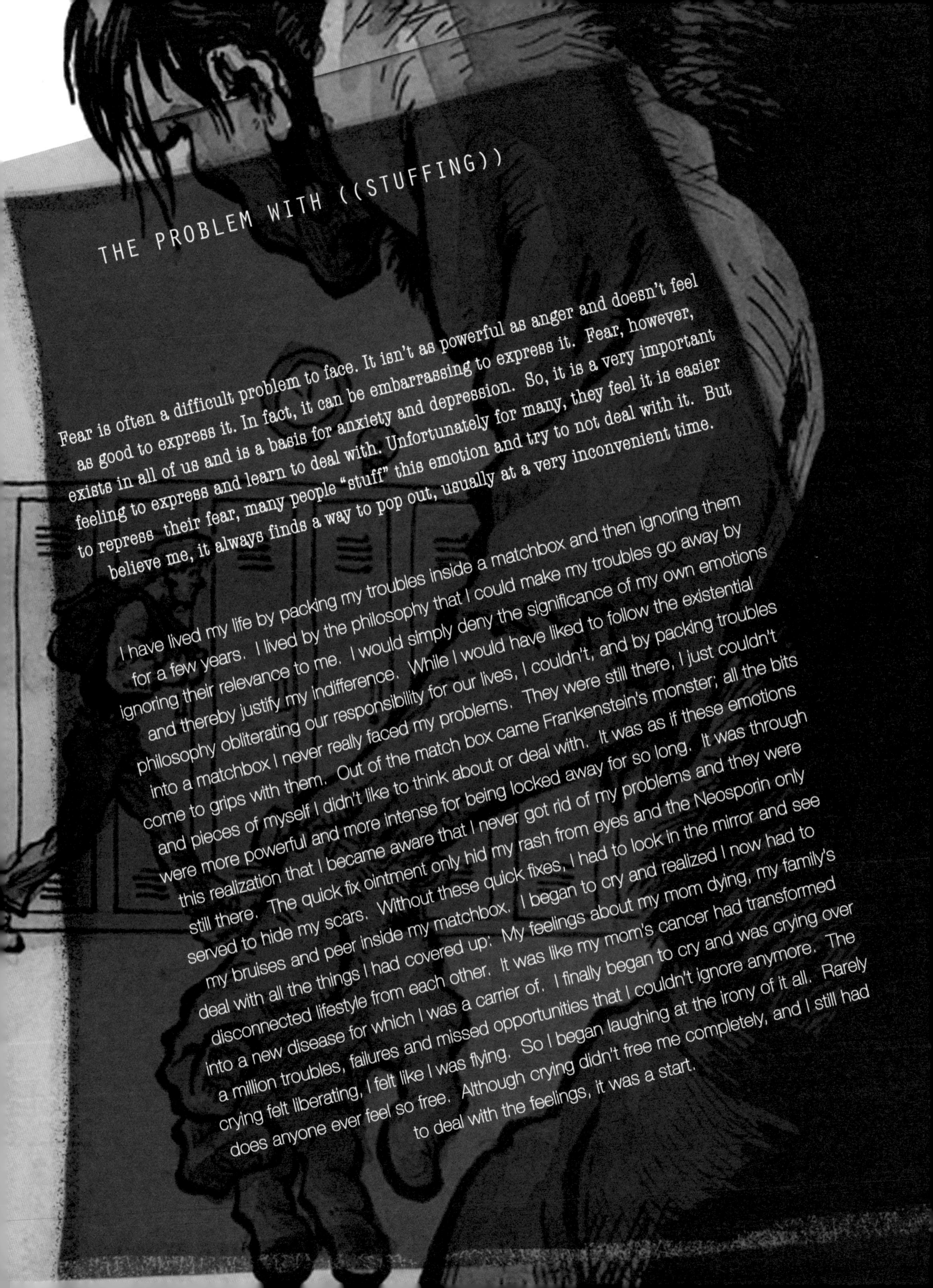

THE PROBLEM WITH ((STUFFING))

Fear is often a difficult problem to face. It isn't as powerful as anger and doesn't feel as good to express it. In fact, it can be embarrassing to express it. Fear, however, exists in all of us and is a basis for anxiety and depression. So, it is a very important feeling to express and learn to deal with. Unfortunately for many, they feel it is easier to repress their fear, many people "stuff" this emotion and try to not deal with it. But believe me, it always finds a way to pop out, usually at a very inconvenient time.

I have lived my life by packing my troubles inside a matchbox and then ignoring them for a few years. I lived by the philosophy that I could make my troubles go away by ignoring their relevance to me. I would simply deny the significance of my own emotions and thereby justify my indifference. While I would have liked to follow the existential philosophy obliterating our responsibility for our lives, I couldn't, and by packing troubles into a matchbox I never really faced my problems. They were still there, I just couldn't come to grips with them. Out of the match box came Frankenstein's monster; all the bits and pieces of myself I didn't like to think about or deal with. It was as if these emotions were more powerful and more intense for being locked away for so long. It was through this realization that I became aware that I never got rid of my problems and they were still there. The quick fix ointment only hid my rash from eyes and the Neosporin only served to hide my scars. Without these quick fixes, I had to look in the mirror and see my bruises and peer inside my matchbox. I began to cry and realized I now had to deal with all the things I had covered up; My feelings about my mom dying, my family's disconnected lifestyle from each other. It was like my mom's cancer had transformed into a new disease for which I was a carrier of. I finally began to cry and was crying over a million troubles, failures and missed opportunities that I couldn't ignore anymore. The crying felt liberating, I felt like I was flying. So I began laughing at the irony of it all. Rarely does anyone ever feel so free. Although crying didn't free me completely, and I still had to deal with the feelings, it was a start.

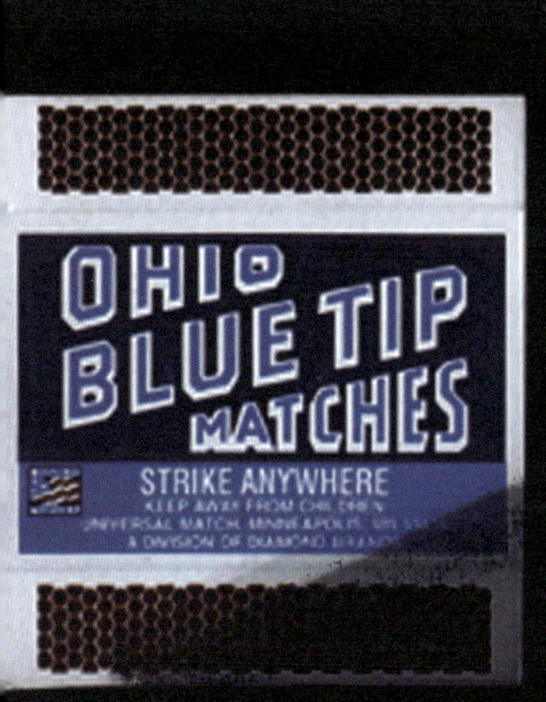

I have had to learn the hard way about my emotions. So here's a quick summary. We must have caution when dealing with our troubles. To some extent they are part of our make up as human beings. So we cannot ignore the validity of their existence or their relevance. However, if we let our pain define us entirely we will not be able to move into the future without letting go of what we've become. My solution is to learn from my troubles and not put them in a matchbox or obsess over them.

In quoting Bryan Tracey,
"obstacles come not to obstruct, but to instruct."
By learning from pain and not
hiding it behind the
laughter we can throw away
most any chance of
Frankenstein
coming out of the closet.
If you can find some way to laugh about your
issues, they will be that much easier to face
and learn
from if they appear funny rather than
menacing. So let go of it and
your troubles rest in peace.

Grady, 18 years old

The cramped quarters of the bus hindered movement as I struggled to get the cellphone from my pocket. It rang once more and I pressed the green "accept call" button. The world around me suddenly went still. Everything dimmed as I heard my father tell me words that I had hoped never to hear. Words that threatened to tear apart my world. "Mom is running a fever." To a normal average person, a fever isn't the best thing to have and it's not fun to be sick. But my mom has cancer. Aggressive, stage four lymphoma – non-curable. She had been going through chemotherapy and was weak.

Her immune system was extremely low, almost non-existent. A fever could easily end her life if medical attention wasn't given to her soon enough. Dad was saying that he didn't know what to do and that she could die any minute. I was scared, sure I was frightened that I might lose my mom forever. Not just my mother, but she had been a real Mom to me; the idea of losing that scared my badly.

I spent the next three days at my grandparents' house feeling all alone and scared. I had no friends to call, no one that really knew or understood the inner struggle I went through. This internal battle over my view of reality…and I was losing.

I only received one phone call from dad. He told me to pray, because it didn't look too good. The rest of my time was spent in the dark clouds of fear and the unknown. I was terrified she might die, and I tried to recall my last words to her. Probably something stupid, not the "I love you Mom, forever and ever" those words that I would want her to leave with. I couldn't see her, speak to her, or even know how she was. Although I kept a good, strong appearance for my younger siblings and grandparents, inside I was a panic-stricken little child, lost in a fear I never knew existed. I remember sitting on the porch swing into the late hours of the night, staring into nothing, thinking nothing only crying soft silent tears.

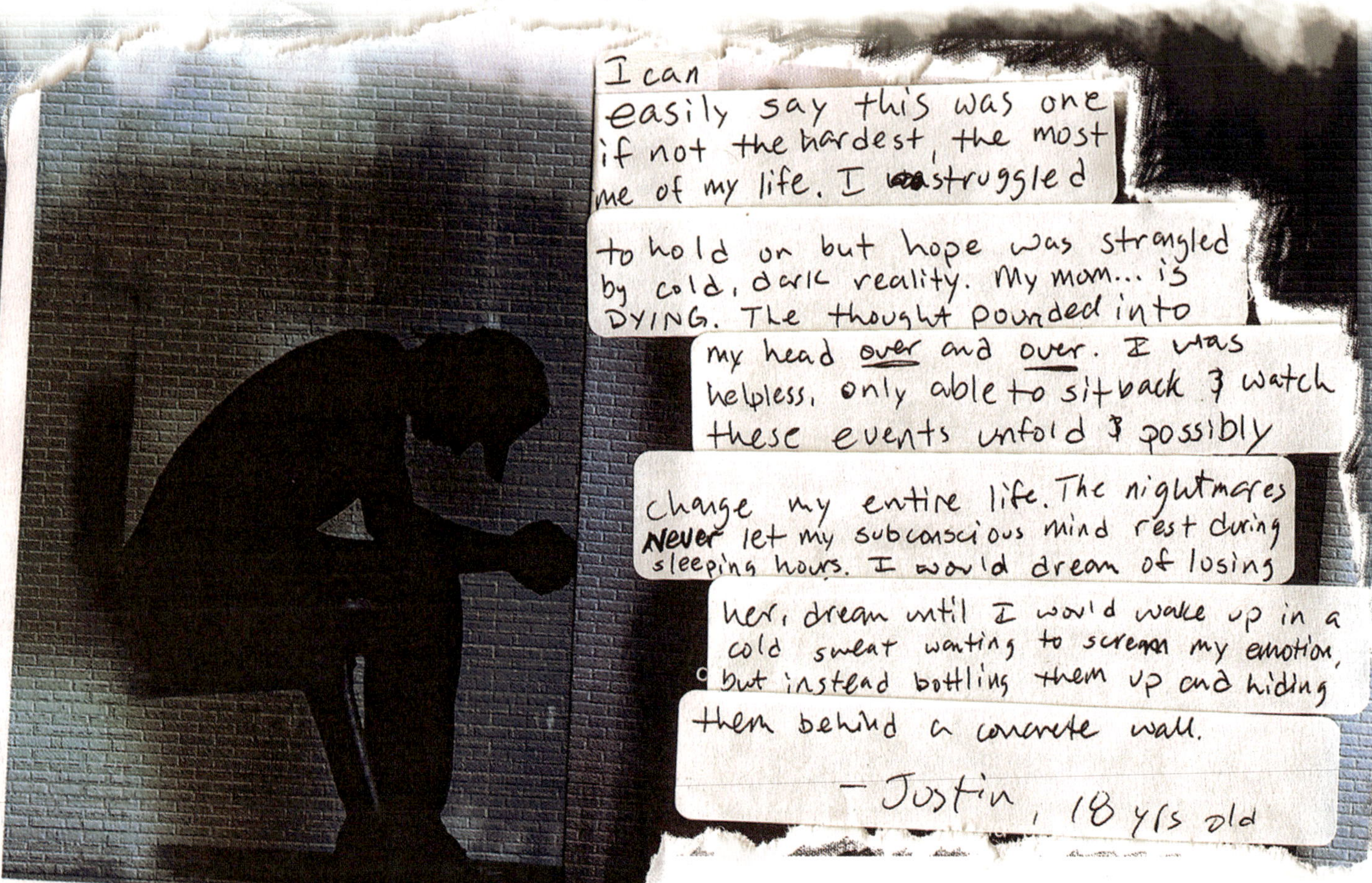

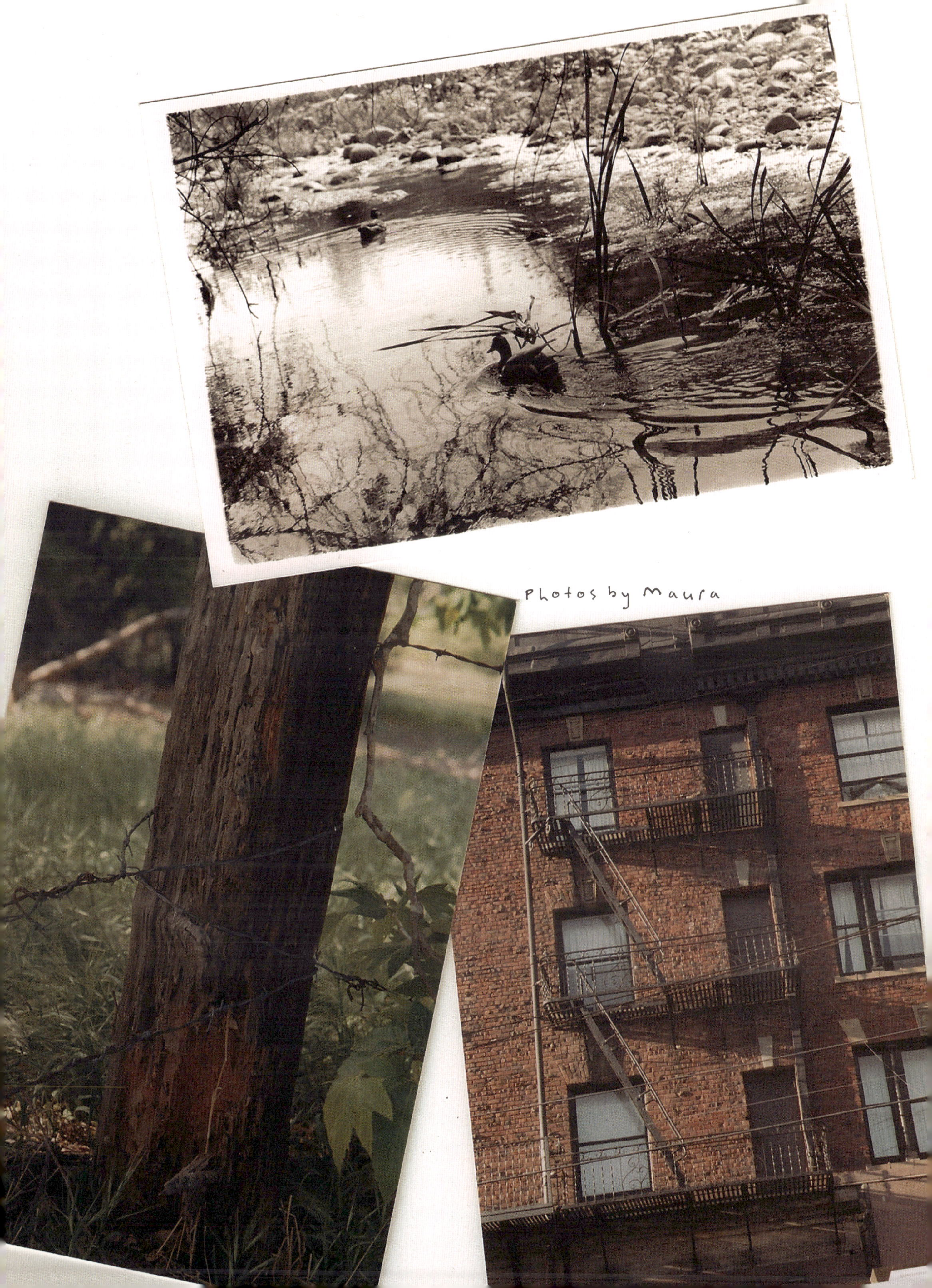

Photos by Maura

Jul. 8th, 2007 at 8:10 PM

Last night I was taking a break from my AP homework, and while my friend was on my computer, and I went outside to sit with my mom by the pool. Before too long she starts talking about what she's going to do if things go south with my dad . . . like sell the house once we all move out, for instance. And honestly, I don't know who is expected to have these kinds of conversations without crying themselves, which I did. She also told about how the one and only time she ever saw my dad cry, throughout their whole marriage, was when he came out of the intensive care unit at the hospital, and the doctors told him his diagnosis/prognosis. She said that his chin just started shaking and that he told her how sorry he was and 'the kids are just babies . . . just babies . . . I'm so sorry."

I have never ever ever ever seen my dad cry, or come even close, and this image just breaks my heart. This whole situation breaks my heart. The hardest part about all of this . . . is feeling like I am just waiting . . . just waiting for the day he dies and all of my misery can hit me full force. I know this probably isn't the best attitude to take on, but consider the fact that out of 33,000 people diagnosed with pancreatic cancer each year, less than 1% manage to beat it completely, and less than 5% live longer then 5 years after they are diagnosed.
THAT IS F*#!ING DEPRESSING!!!

Do you know how much I HATE watching people slowly kill themselves but living on like it's nothing?! How much I HATE knowing the fact that even though my dad doesn't drink, smoke, and works hard to take care of himself, he still has to sit at home feeling sick all the time, breaking out with worse acne then I have ever had, and puking everyday thanks to his chemo THAT PROBABLY WON'T EVEN WORK. Life f*#!ing sucks. That is all there is to it. If there is anybody who doesn't deserve it, it is my dad. It really is.

Thursday, August 09, 2007 11:51 PM

When tomorrow starts without me, and I'm not there to see; If the sun should rise and find your eyes all filled with tears for me; I wish so much you wouldn't cry the way you did today, While thinking of the many things we didn't get to say. I know how much you love me, as much as I love you,
And each time you think of me,
I know you'll miss me, too;
But when tomorrow starts without me, please try to understand, That an angel came and called my name and took me by the hand, And said my place was ready in heaven far above, And that I'd have to leave behind all those I dearly love.
But as I turned to walk away, a tear fell from my eye,
For all my life, I'd always thought I didn't want to die.
I had so much to live for and so much yet to do, It seemed almost impossible that I was leaving you. I thought of all the yesterdays, the good ones and the bad,
I thought of all the love we shared and all the fun we had. If I could relive yesterday, I thought, just for a while, I'd say good-bye and kiss you and maybe see your smile.

Miranda's Blog

But then I fully realized that this could never be, For emptiness and memories would take place of me. And when I thought of worldly things that I'd miss tomorrow, I thought of you, and when I did, my heart was filled with sorrow. But when I walked through heaven's gates, I felt so at home. When God looked down and smiled at me, from His great golden throne, He said, "This is eternity and all I've promised you, Today for life on Earth is past but here it starts anew. I promise no tomorrow, but today will always last, And since each day's the same day, there's no longing for the past. But you have been so faithful, so trusting and so true, Though there were times you did some things you knew you shouldn't do. But you have been forgiven and now at last you're free. So won't you take my hand and share my life with me?" So when tomorrow starts without me, don't think we're far apart, For every time you think of me, I'm right here in your heart.
David M. Romano

This poem made me cry.

Sep. 3rd, 2007 at 4:23 PM

Yesterday was pretty crappy. I tried really hard to get out of that stupid BBQ and it turned into a huge argument with my dad. Basically, he blew up at me, not for any real reason I think, because I didn't deserve it, but because he's stressed . . . and who would blame him? Anyway, some of the stuff he said to me was pretty crappy, and of course my brother has to jump in, against me, and instead of my dad telling him to mind his own business . . . he agreed. Whatever. I was crying for quite a few hours so then I had a headache ALL day as a result, and not one apology . . . but some things you just have to get over I suppose.

Sep. 6th, 2007 at 8:37 PM

Maybe if I'm perfectly together on the outside, I'll be alright on the inside too.

Sorry if I've been a b*#!h lately. It sounds stupid but I kinda can't help it.

Sep. 19th, 2007 at 8:42 PM

This past week has been a confusing set of emotions for me. On the one hand, I'm really really thankful about my Dad's CT scans and knowing that he will be around that much longer. On the other hand, I still wish he could just be better . . . and everytime I think about how hard and unfair all this is, and what my life will be like without him, I feel like I'm going to break down. I also feel like I've grown up really fast in a very small amount of time, and part of me is proud of myself and my new priorities, but part of me wishes it was still easy to be so breezy and relate to things my friends talk about and feel. I also feel alone, and I don't know what I want, and I KNOW that I'm pushing people away, but I'm still upset when they don't come

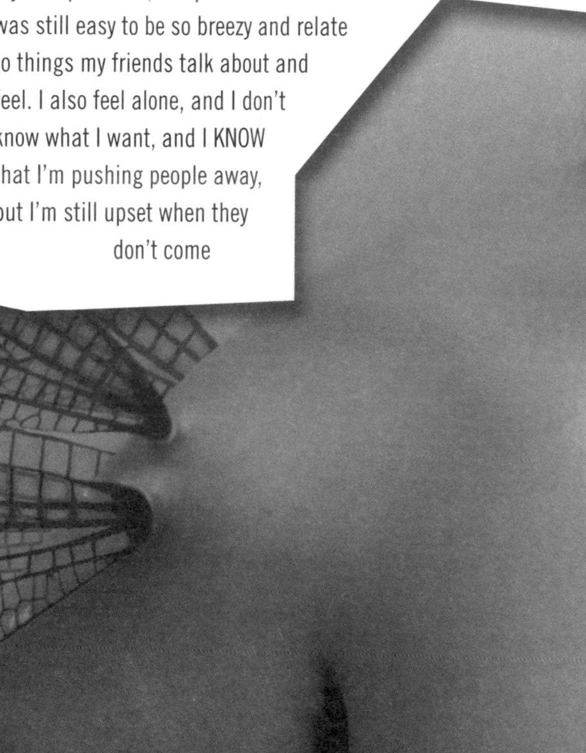

back. I don't know if I'm doing this because it's truely justified (I've matured or they've been crappy and it's not worth my time) or if I'm doing this to reduce emotional ties, and limit who has the power to break my heart. I think it's the latter, but I don't know how to stop. Consider me officially damaged.

Sep. 25th, 2007 at 3:12 PM

Ok. Time to stop being depressed. I don't want to be depressed I just don't know how. I should clean my room. Start there. Ugh. It's just hard. Don't know what is wrong with me, seriously. Tomorrow is a minimum day, so I can ease my way in I guess? In my current state, I don't know how I will do anything.

Oct. 14th, 2007 at 3:07 PM

I really need to pull myself together.

December 5th 2007 10:30 PM

"It's like you're empty, you're not even here anymore . . ." and the saddest part is that it's true.

Thursday, December 13, 2007 10:04 PM

So as most of you know my dad's health is declining, and last Monday his scans results confirmed that there are more spots on his liver. Right now he is on the list to do a biopsy but it would be a miracle if those spots didn't mean that his cancer has metastisized. This puts radiation out of the picture completely. He has also lost a lot of weight recently (anybody who's seen him can testify to that) and he's on pain meds all the time now because he is hurting so bad. The signs are all there, and realistically, my dad is probably facing the end of his life -something we're all having a really, really difficult time coming to terms with.

I'm not writing this to gain sympathy or attention, but simply to say that this next semester I'm taking time for myself and my family. I love my dad very very much and I don't ever want to feel like I'm not doing the things I should be doing right now. I haven't been a good friend for a long time now, nor have I been very fair to any of you, and I know this isn't an excuse but please realize the things I'm dealing with right now.

This is topic that is very hard for me to talk about or write about without getting upset, but there are things I want to get out to all you guys that I don't have the emotional capacity to explain over and over. Number one, like I said, I'm sorry I haven't been the best person lately and please forgive me and understand me for that. Number two, I don't want to talk about it, because I'll get upset and the rest of my day is ruined. Just trust me when I say it's bad and unless I bring it up I don't want to go into huge details because it breaks my heart.

And lastly, and most importantly, I am taking time for myself and my family this semester. In the future PLEASE just accept when I say I don't want to hang out tonight, and don't push it because it's hard enough for me to do already. This is because I want to spend time with my dad and my family while I still have the chance, and I don't want my best friends running around thinking that I'm just being lame. I love you guys and I know it's stupid of me to have to even ask to be left alone on this issue, but I feel it's important that everyone knows what's up. I don't see any reason that anybody would get mad for what I'm doing but all the same this is the decision I'm making and I'm sorry I won't be the same party girl I've been, but this is how it's got be right now until something changes. Like I said, I love you guys.

Dec. 22nd, 2007 at 1:04 AM

Looking back at the past few months, I feel like I'm just sinking in a hole, and occassionally I make progress but for the most part I just get worse. I'm STILL dealing with depression and being a bad friend and smoking more than I should. I don't understand why, for all my trying, I don't get better.

As my dad gets sicker I feel worse and considering I don't ever see it getting better, I don't ever see myself getting happy either. And it sucks.

Tonight I went to this service with a friend at his church, and oh my god did it give me a lot to think about. Lately I've been thinking a lot about God and what happens when a person dies, because for so long I just haven't believed in anything . . . not God or any kind of afterlife, but that's such a hard view to maintain when I think about what is going to happen to my dad and the people I love, eventually. I'm trying really hard to believe in something, in some kind of God or some kind of heaven, because I think it would really help me with the way I'm feeling, it's just so hard when you've believed something else for so long. The things they all said tonight sounded so nice, but a lot of it just seemed just plain ridiculous to me. That's a terrible thing to write but that's how I feel. I'm trying really hard to make this work, I just don't know where to begin, and I'm afraid.

I'm so damn tired. I'm exhausted.

Tuesday, January 22, 2008 9:25 PM

My dad is turning yellow again. I can see it in the whites of his eyes. I told him and he said, "That's just too damn bad." I don't know what that means but I don't like the sound of it. He is sooo tired, all of the time now. It breaks my heart to watch. I wish I just had more time.

Wednesday, January 23, 2008 10:45 PM

I'm miserable right now. My dad is in the emergency room with a temperature of 102. Hopefully he will feel better after some antibiotics but I'm scared shitless. I don't know what the future is going to hold and I'm scared I could lose him any day now. I don't know what to expect, but from what I hear and read nothing I see is good. He's tired all the time and seems like he spends most of his time now asleep. His eyes are yellow again, his liver is out of control, and I'm going crazy with worry. I hate seeing him like this and none of this is fair. My dad hasn't ever done anything to deserve this, and I can confidently say that he's the best person I've ever known. I'm having trouble functioning with everything I do. I just want him to feel better again. I just want another good day.

Wednesday, January 16, 2008 5:40 PM

Seems like people forget it's ok to be sad too.

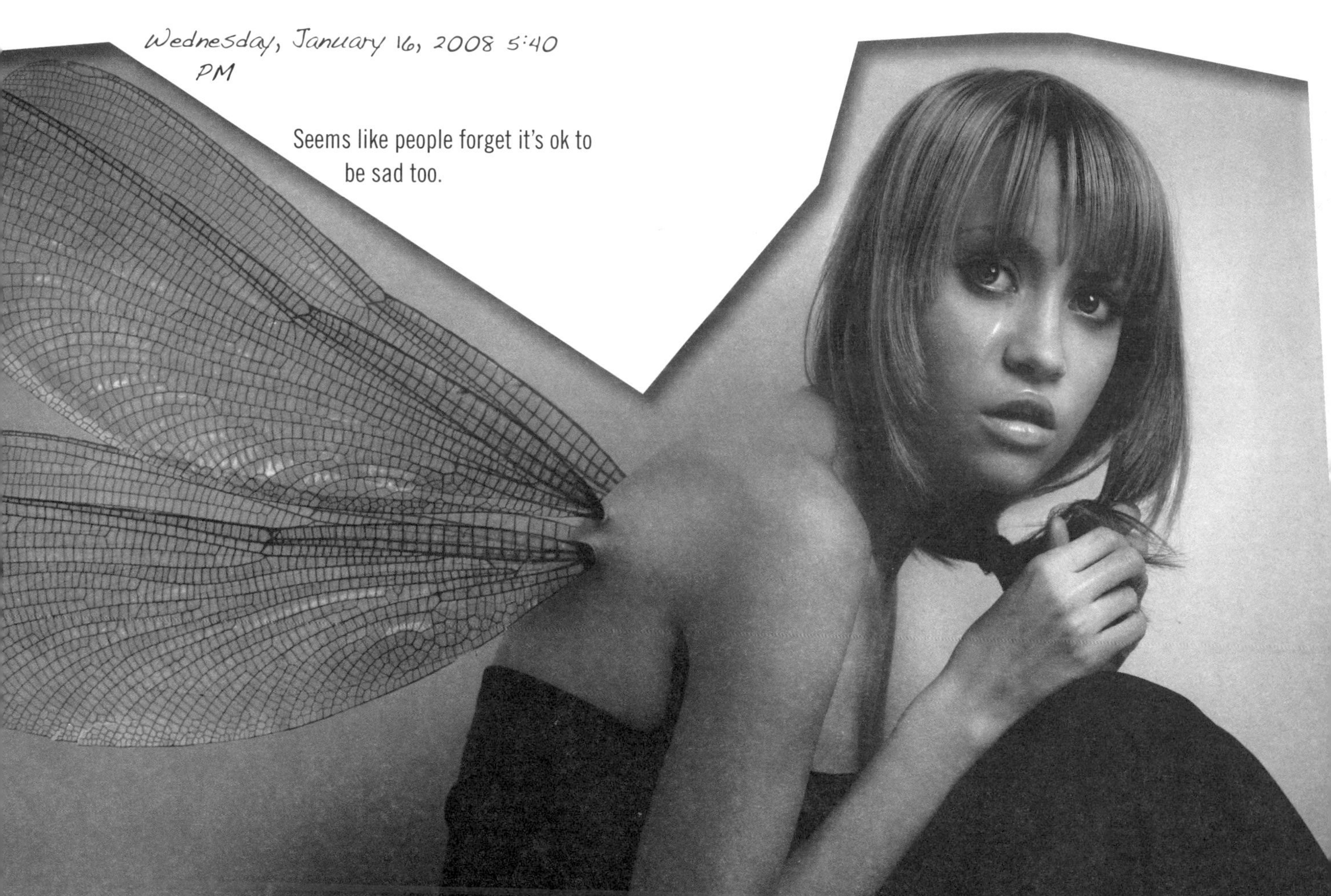

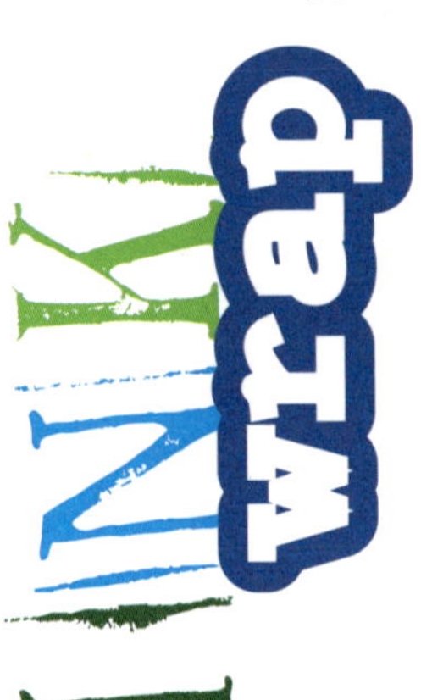

FEAR may probably be the most difficult emotion for you to deal with during your parent's cancer or death. As a teen you are not necessarily equipped right now with a lot of "insight" into yourself and your feelings, this won't come until you are well into your 20s. This makes it an almost impossible task to for you to be able to regularly express feelings of vulnerability such as fear. You may have learned through the years to become a "stuffer" of your emotions, as you strive to fit in, blend in and to never, ever be noticed in a "bad" or "awkward" way.

So, if suddenly you are dealing with a parent who has lost her hair, or it is getting around your community that your family needs "help,"…. well this can be social suicide. It's embarrassing to have this type of attention. **YOU MAY ALSO FEAR WHAT SORT OF CHANGES ARE AHEAD OF YOU.** How will your parent's cancer or death affect you? What responsibilities are you now going to have? How will this impact your day-to-day life? You may fear losing your "childhood" and unfortunately this may be your reality if you are facing your parents cancer diagnosis or death.

You may have perfected the "I'm fine" mantra when asked by your parents "how are you doing?" regarding their cancer diagnosis. The reality, however, is that you probably are not "fine," and sometimes you don't even realize that you are not fine. Support groups and individual therapy can be helpful for you to talk about and deal with your feelings. You might be reluctant to talk to your parents about your feelings. Maybe this is due to the natural *"secrecy"* that teens have, but it can also be due to a desire to "protect" your parent from your feelings. The problem is when you don't feel as if you have someone to talk to or can discuss your feelings with, this can cause you to feel anxious or even depressed. This anxiety can come from rational and irrational fears that you may be facing. How can you tell if you are having normal worries of if your worry has turned into anxiety.

HERE ARE SOME SIGNS OF ANXIETY:

- Excessive worrying, ruminating or obsessing
- Nervous habits (such as nail biting, picking at your skin, etc.)
- Irritability
- Impaired concentration
- Feeling restless or on edge
- Self-consciousness and insecurity
- Heart palpitations, butterflies in your stomach

By talking through your feelings you can sort through the fears and feel more confident in your coping abilities and relieve your feelings of anxiety. You can also feel like you are not alone in dealing with this adversity in your life.

- Lynnette

THE RULE FOR OVERCOMING FEAR IS TO HEAD RIGHT INTO IT.

ANONYMOUS

"Every guy wants to be a "macho man," it's perfectly natural. I know that personally because I try to keep a tough image. Playing football and lacrosse, this sort of a reputation is expected; don't cry and don't show emotion, these are the unspoken rules. And this is the image that I keep, but it does not mean that I don't show my emotions, express my feelings, and or even occasionally cry when the time is right.

Your close family and friends already know the "real" you and the feelings and emotions that come along with that, and they have always loved you so there should be no fear in expressing them. Dealing with a parent with cancer, or a parent with any illness, is an extremely difficult and emotional time. The emotions that you, as a guy, feel are O.K. and perfectly natural; even "tough guys" can cry. If you are not comfortable with sharing openly right away, express your feelings with your parents, then close buddies, and slowly work toward being open all the time with your emotions. Just remember that it is healthy to express your feelings in the grieving process, and having feeling does not make you any less of a "macho man."

Plus as a final thought, girls love a strong man that can show his emotions too; it's a good thing to know! Just be true to yourself, everyone expresses their feelings in a different way, just be sure that you do express them in some way, shape or form."

Cole, 17 years old

A tough reputation does not at all mean that you have to deny your feelings or even pretend like you don't have any. All a reputation is, is a mask that people that don't truly know you see.

Awkward, Pitiful Questions

Has someone ever asked you if your mom could take you to your friend's house or the movies or anywhere? Has someone ever laid a "your momma joke" on you? Well, being an exceptionally social person in a have fun go-hang-out high school world is difficult with just one parent. When I was 5 years old, on the 17th of November in 1997; on this day, my mom fought and lost to breast cancer.

When my dad came home that night, my brother (9) and my sister (7) and I all learned of our mom's death. My sister and brother suddenly in tears and I didn't understand why. I asked myself, "Why is this so bad?", and "It's not that bad."

That was me, ten years ago in shock. Over the next few days I carried on as normal, except everything we ate was prepared and given to us to eat from friends and neighbors. I was still in shock. When the funeral came around, I was over the shock, the pain had set in and I finally understood why people were bringing us dinner and brother, my sister, and my dad were crying. At the funeral, I bawled like there was no tomorrow.

Usually I do not like to tell people that my mom died from breast cancer. I don't like to tell people because when I do, people go "awww, I'm sorry" and then a minute later they don't care or even remember. That fakeass pity disgusts me. It's not always the pity that gets me; it's the pain. The pain of someone laughing at a "your momma joke" aimed at you. The pain of recalling my mom's funeral. The pain of life. By Conor, age 15

USE THIS PAGE

if wishes were

- anonymous

If wishes were as **voices** are
and could be heard as clearly
then **you** would hear
unspoken words from my heart -
whispered **softly**

"Love, you are as a **dream**
to me those peaceful plays
of the mind. **You carry me** to
secret places where reality
and fantasy entwine"

If you see yourself as
an **opened** book
Then judge me not unfairly
My pages, as **yours**,
shall never speak
Except when read sincerely

My Dad is a Yellow Man

My dad was a yellow man, literally. Since Christmas he'd lost so much weight he was unrecognizable, and after all the tests and biopsies, we still didn't know what was wrong. All we knew was that there was a tumor blocking his gall bladder duct, but that it was benign and a whipple procedure could fix everything up. It was April 1st, and his surgery was scheduled early the next morning.

My mom spent her nights crying. Dad told me that she was just being a little irrational, talking herself into believing it was cancer and that she'd end up alone in a giant house with two teenagers to raise. He told me that he was going to be ok.

He called me back to his room, and I sat down on the couch across from him, wondering what it was he had to say to all of us, myself and my two brothers, that could be so important. He explained to me that he would be okay, but that surgery was surgery and there were things he wanted to say.

"This is probably the only time you will hear me do this, but . . ."

He told me that he was glad to see I was doing well since my recent break up with my boyfriend, and that I could handle the death of our dog just fine too. He reminded me that I didn't need a man in my life to make me happy, and that I was beautiful and smart and that I could truly exceed in whatever it is that I wanted to do with my life. He took the time to describe just how smart my brothers were too, and asked me to be a little nicer to them if I could, and he would say the same to them. He told me to try and be more understanding of my mom, and be nice to her too.

My dad is not an open man. He doesn't tell you how he feels, he just simply shows you. And when he said that I'd never hear it again, he wasn't kidding. In my head I said, "Thanks Dad. But tomorrow you're going to be ok, and this will all go away."

I walked out of that room in a daze, realizing for the first time how scared I was. That night I couldn't sleep. I had horrible nightmares: over and over the doctors telling me that my dad had cancer, that he was going to die, and there was nothing they could do. I screamed and cried and kept asking, "What the hell am I supposed to do now?! This happens to other people, not to my dad . . . how am I supposed to go on without him?"

I woke up at 4:30 in the morning, feeling relieved; the sense of doom pushed to the very back of my mind, and today, my dad would be okay. Today, my dad didn't have cancer.

When I waved my dad off to the hospital, I told him that I just wanted to say goodbye to him. I didn't mention my nightmares or how scared I was, but he took it as a nice gesture and went on his way. Eventually I fell back asleep, in an attempt to make time go by a little faster, waking up to daylight. Eager for more news, I called my mom multiple times to try and figure out what was going on, each time her annoyance increasing, telling me that she knew nothing yet.

Finally, around noon, she told me that she was having my best friend's mother come pick us up, my younger brother Shane and myself, to take us to the hospital. Somewhere in my head I asked why, if it was good news, she wouldn't just tell me over the phone, but I rationalized and decided that her voice wasn't shaking or breaking, and we should be at the hospital anyway. Everything was still okay.

At the hospital we met my grandpa in the elevator, coming back from a funeral, on his way to hear the news alongside my brother and myself. My mom had secured a little backroom that we could use all day if we wanted, but I could tell by the way my dad's friends and coworkers cleared the room that it wasn't good. I could tell by my grandma's red eyes and the tissue in her hand, that very soon I would be crying too.

And then I was. I can remember my mom telling us that they had opened him up and all they could do was rearrange some ducts to make him more comfortable, but couldn't do anything for his tumor; that pancreatic cancer was bad and we probably didn't have long. I can remember my grandma telling me that it's okay to cry, and our goal was to keep him healthy until the next big race in Mexico, then until my graduation, and then until Shane's graduation. I can remember my grandpa exclaiming, "Oh Jesus!" and Shane just sitting there, taking it all in. Mostly, in my head, I can just remember thinking, my nightmare has come true.

I sat in that room for a long time, wondering how this could happen to us. My dad wasn't a drinker, he wasn't a smoker, and maybe he'd eaten a little too much red meat but that wasn't something that was deserving of cancer. Over and over in my head I played out how everything had happened. When he first got sick, that Christmas day, experiencing an odd lurch in his stomach, I don't think the first thought in any of our heads was, "Oh God, this could kill him." We just assumed he would eventually get better, you always assume somebody will eventually get better . . .

When my dad woke up, my mom and I were the first ones who went back to visit him. He was so tiny and frail in that hospital bed, hooked up to all his tubes and drugs, that it was really hard for me to hold back tears. He heard my sniffling with a concerned look on his face he

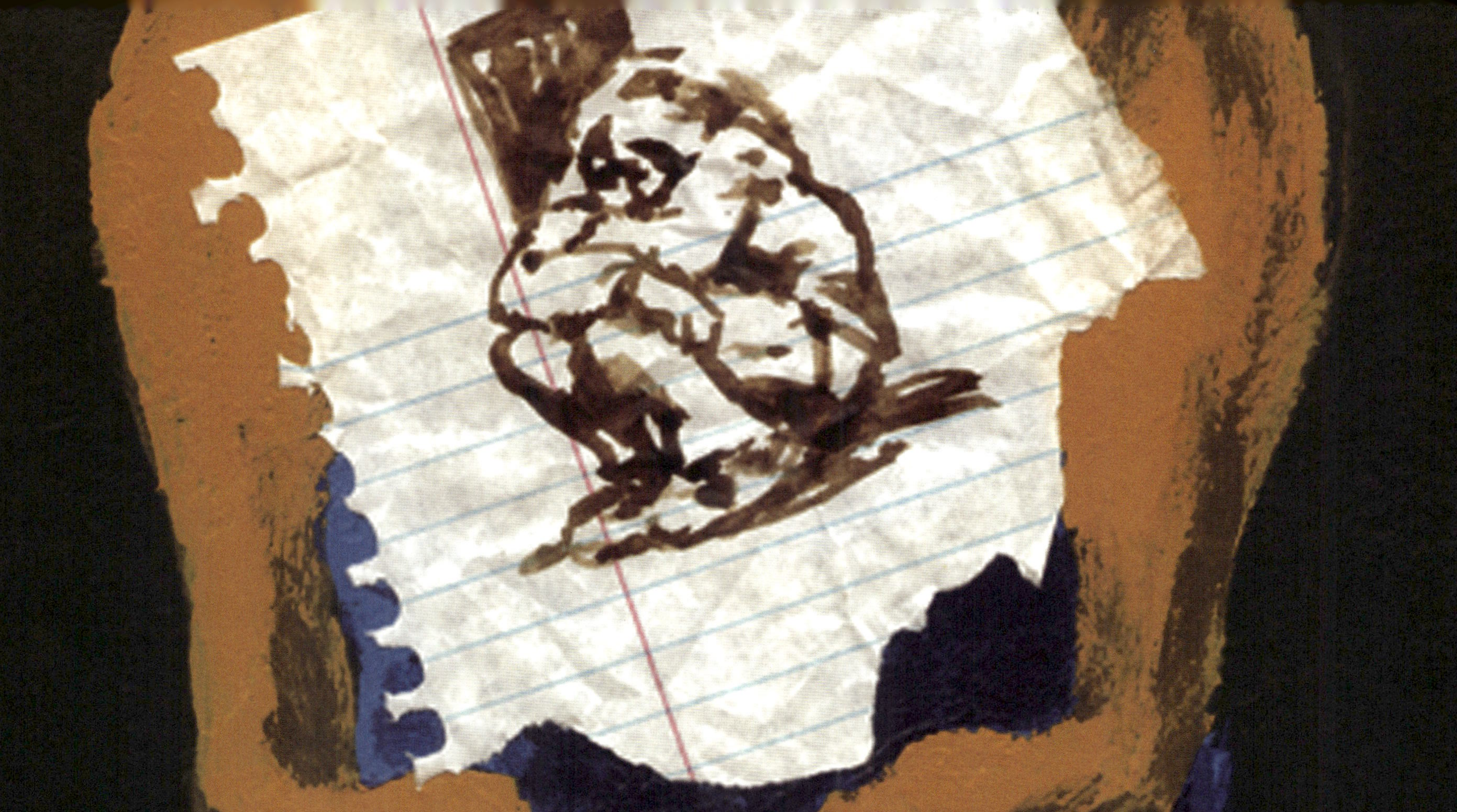

asked if I was ok. I assured him that I was, and after double checking, he closed his eyes again.

Here he is, straight out of a major surgery and facing two more weeks in the hospital, and he's more concerned about whether or not I'M okay! At this point he was completely unaware of his diagnosis, and even if we had told him right then, he wouldn't have remembered. My dad was just happy to wake up, glad to be able to open his eyes again.

Since we could only go back to his room in twos, and since there were so many people there to see him, it probably took about an hour before he went through them all. My grandpa came out saying, "My god! George is back there doing stand up comedy!" Everyone walked out of that room smiling, and when my mom and I went back there to say goodbye, he sat there rolling his eyes in disbelief telling us that his brother had been making fun of him, saying he wouldn't remember any of their conversation. When Mom in fact confirmed that he wouldn't, he became genuinely upset.

"Ok Ginni, since I can't remember any of it, there's some important stuff I need you to remember for me . . ."

Even days later, after he'd learned what was going on, we never saw him upset. He simply said, "I beat it when I was 18, and I'll beat it now." He continued to keep everybody ELSE entertained, and eventually I realized, that even through all of this, the worst days of my life, all we could do was make the best of it, and that is enough.

Pray for another good day,
and that is enough.

Miranda, age 17

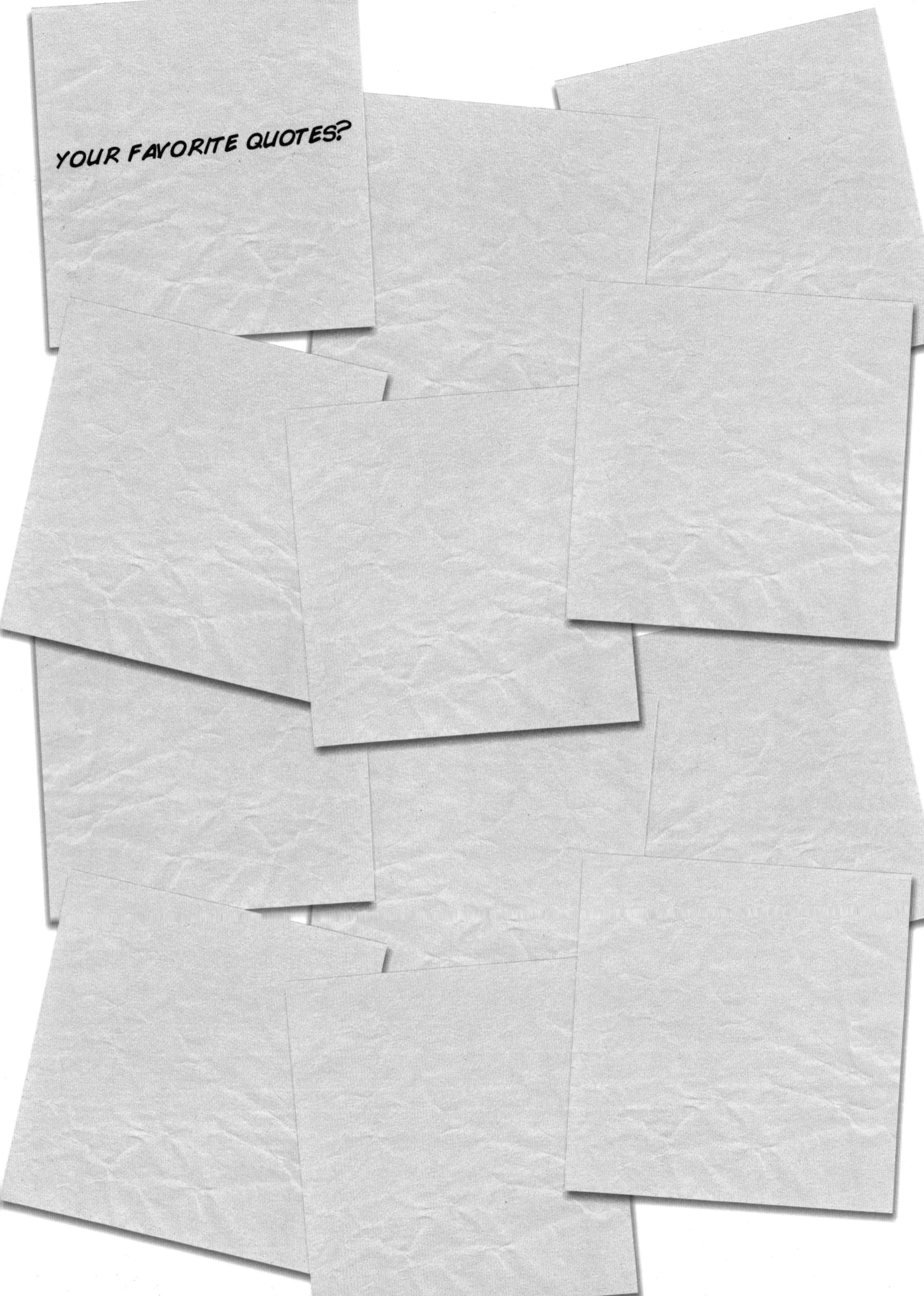
YOUR FAVORITE QUOTES?

SHRINK wrap

Sadness is a very difficult feeling for most teens. Much of your sadness may be covered up in layers of anger. Anger is just a more acceptable, more "in control" feeling than sadness. It may be difficult to discern if you're feeling normal teen sullenness or if you are feeling more reclusive and irritable than usual. It is important to discern the difference between normal sadness and depression. It is normal to experience sadness during your parent's cancer diagnosis. However, if the sadness becomes more than melancholy and begins to interfere with your day to day life, this may be depression. Here are some of the basic signs and symptoms of depression:

1. Loss of interest in normal daily activities, not wanting to go to school.
2. Depressed mood, feeling hopeless or helpless.
3. Needing too much sleep or not being able to sleep at all.
4. Over eating or not being able to eat.
5. Crying all the time.
6. Impaired ability to concentrate
7. Restless, agitated, irritable and easily annoyed.
8. Low self-esteem, feeling worthless and having excessive guilt.
9. Thoughts of death, dying or suicide.

- Lynnette

When I was a junior in high school, my mom was diagnosed with breast cancer in October... Which, incidentally, is also breast cancer awareness month.

Funny how that works, huh?

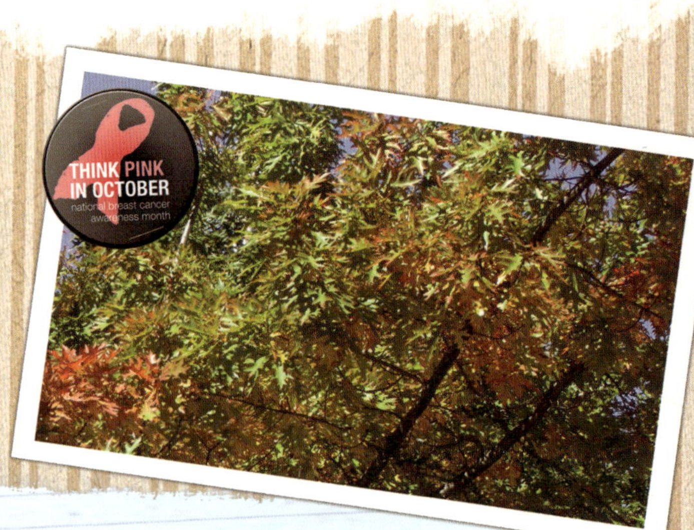

I was, not surprisingly, completely floored when my dad told me.

I'm just like everyone else – I knew cancer is out there, but come on, there's no way it can enter my life….wrong. The next day at school was probably the worst day of my life. I was hesitant to tell my three best friends, because it would make my mom's condition too real. Even now I smile remembering how angry my friends were that I didn't tell them immediately. Not really angry, but you know, indignant. But after I told them, I didn't tell anyone else I knew. It had been hard enough to be sobbing in front of my best friends; I couldn't help keeping it to myself from then on.

I guess short-term, holding it in was great. I didn't have to deal with the "oh-my-gosh-that-sucks-I'm sorry's", or people thinking they had to go easy on poor old Lydia because her mom's sick. I mean, please. But, looking back now, keeping my secret all bottled up was probably pretty detrimental to the healing process. For almost two years, I didn't tell anyone I was close to about my mom not boyfriends, new friends teacher….Nope. I had a lot of issues that weren't even related to cancer then, and I think my unreleased feelings were kind of poisoning my life, attracting negativity.

But, I remember now that the moment I let go of my secrecy about my mom, it became a lot easier to deal with the fact that cancer has touched my life. I'm not sad about it anymore, I just deal with it as a part of my life. By releasing my problem, I made room in my heart for feelings I hadn't had before. I think that growth is a complicated thing. Our body grows steadily over time, but the soul grows by leaps and bounds. When I decided to let go of my secrecy, the capacity of my soul got bigger, more mature and overnight I made a monumental step in becoming a woman. So, as corny as it is when someone tells you holding it in is wrong, they're unfortunately right.

You may want to tell them to shove their self-help talk up their, well, you know, but take it in stride and try to understand it's the right thing.

Lydia 19 yrs old

Friends suck, they are the greatest gifts outside of my family and talents. Its funny being such a big gift, only gives them more power and leverage to bring and cause pain. The irony goes even deeper when the realization is that the friends who give us this pain are what teens build their lives around. It's a risk, one we are always willing to take and one we are never willing to learn from. It's like digging our own grave. Of course, what would the world be like without that pain that only a friend can give? In reality it is that pain that we use to reevaluate ourselves and push ourselves to greater aspirations. It is in this gift of pain that friends have their most value. When they unknowingly give it, they are more than ready to help take it away. But before they take it away, they bring ourselves into question and force us to redefine everything. Then once we reach that unique insight which pain gives us, our friends help to lift the remnants of that pain and we, as a person are all the better for it.

A true friend is the one who offers nothing more than friendship and understanding. A true friend will ask me what I need and then help with that, no matter how inconvenient it may be. At times, the role of a true friend is ambivalent and sure you may feel they are overstepping their boundaries, but it isn't done with malevolence. When they do hurt us it only brings us that shock of pain that reawakens us to reality and out of our sometimes self-centered world.

Grady, age 18

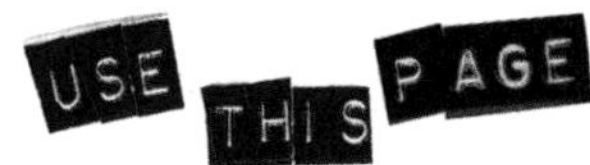
USE THIS PAGE

from the French word, rapprocher (ra-pro-chay) meaning "to bring together"

In a teen's world, your friends are your life. This is the development process of *rapprochement*, as you separate from your parents and join your peers, your friends. It is no wonder then that after a parent is diagnosed with cancer, a teen will flee to their friends and only make rare appearances at home. A problem you may face is that although you want to be with your friends, you also don't want to stand out as being "different." You may not want to talk to your friends about your home life and your parent's illness. So, you may hang out with your friends, carrying the heavy burden of your parent's illness and keeping that secret from those you feel are your ultimate support. Carrying this burden and secret can cause great anxiety, if you are unaware of this anxiety and how to take care of it you may find yourself turning to drugs and alcohol as a way to numb the anxious feelings and "think" this helps you have more control over your emotions. Drugs and alcohol are never the solution. They only become an additional problem that you will someday have to deal with. They also just mask the problems of depression and anxiety actually making them both worse in the long run.

IT IS IMPORTANT TO TALK TO YOUR FRIENDS ABOUT WHAT IS GOING ON. Even if you don't think they really "get" it, it will still help to talk about your situation. They just might surprise you. It may also be frustrating at times listening to your friends talk about their menial problems when you are now dealing with life and death situations. Don't be afraid to let your friends know when you need a little extra support. There will undoubtedly come a time when they will need you too.

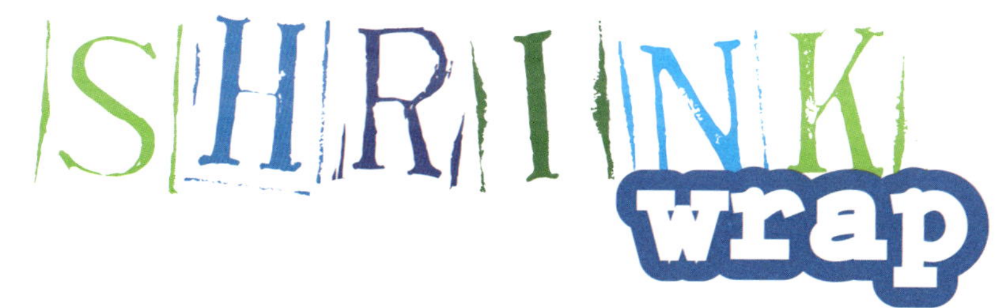

As annoying as it is, it is important for your parents to be aware of your friends and who you are hanging around with. Although it is difficult at times, your parents will probably still enforce their house rules and want you continue to do chores and homework. These boundaries are actually useful and will help ease the anxiety you might be feeling.

This is also a time when support groups are great because you will realize you are not alone and it will give you exposure to friends that you can feel "normal" around and not feel as though they have to keep secrets from. These friends in group will really "get" what you are going through. Individual counseling can also be helpful during this time. A therapist that is experienced in working with teens can give you an ally and someone to talk to about issues that you don't think you can address with your parents.

- Lynnette

School, it's one of those things you have to do, right? However, going to school can be really hard when your parent has cancer, and long, long after that too.

When my Dad was diagnosed with cancer, I found it really, really difficult to go to school. I would take "stress days." Basically ditch days with Mom's consent. You might be saying, hey, what's so bad about that? Day off school without a truancy? This "one day" of excused absence may seem innocent, but wait until you let it stick around enough for it to come back and punch you down. You fall, hard.

And we all know that when you fall it takes time to get back up, right? After my Dad passed away, I was still taking those "stress days." The worst part of all of this was that my Mom let me skip school and stay at home wasting away.
Two and a half years later, as I write this, I still seem to find multiple excuses for not going to school. At this point in my life I am face down on the cold hard floor struggling to get up and find my balance. Sound fun? It isn't!

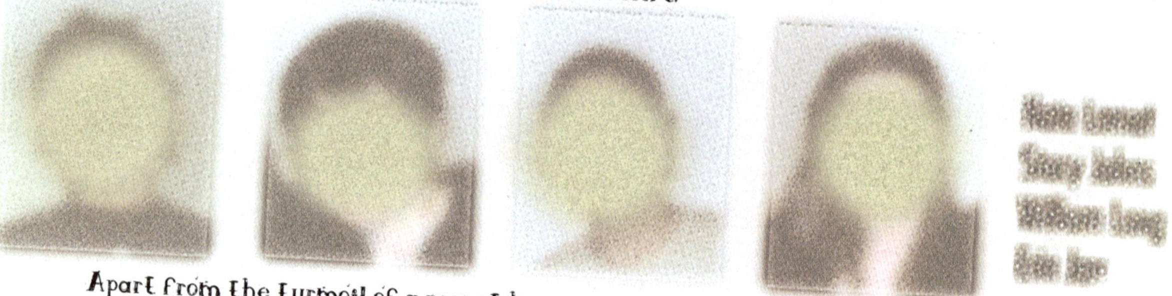

Apart from the turmoil of a parent having cancer, or dying from it, who needs or wants for that matter, to worry about school? Although skipping school seems like the easiest and smartest choice for you right now, believe me, it's not. Even if you just go to school and get the homework and get that little mark next to your name saying that you showed up, it's still way better than sitting at home watching soaps and wallowing in your grief. You may feel ostracized and embarrassed because you are unique and you're standing out and you are under scrutiny from those around you.

Erika,
age 15

MY ALARM CLOCK GOES OFF OR MORE LIKELY MY MOM IS YELLING AND NAGGING ME TO GET UP. I FEEL PARALYZED ALMOST. WHY LEAVE THE WARMTH AND SAFETY OF MY COZY BED TO FACE THE PRESSURES OF SCHOOL? THERE'S JUST NO ANSWER. I FEEL WHY DO I HAVE TO GO THROUGH THE NORMAL PRESSURE OF MY CHANGING LIFE AS A TEENAGER AND HIGH SCHOOL STUDENT HOMEWORK, TESTS, PEER PRESSURE, FRIENDS, BOYS, AND SO ON WHILE GRIEVING FOR MY FATHER? IT'S JUST NOT FAIR, SO I DESERVE NOT TO HAVE TO GO TO SCHOOL. THE HOMEWORK AND TESTS AND REPORTS SEEM TO BECOME SO INSIGNIFICANT AFTER LOSING MY FATHER FOREVER WHO HAD PLAYED SUCH A MAJOR ROLE IN MY LIFE. I BEGIN NOT TO BE ABLE TO BEAR TO LISTEN TO THE PETTY PROBLEMS AND COMMENTS OF MY FRIENDS. IT'S SO UNFAIR THAT THEY DON'T UNDERSTAND AND NEVER REALLY WILL. IT'S UNFAIR THAT THEY DON'T KNOW WHAT TO SAY, SO THEY DON'T SAY ANYTHING AT ALL. BUT I KNOW THERE'S NOTHING I CAN CHANGE ABOUT THAT. I JUST FEEL LIKE CURLING UP IN A BALL AND SLEEPING AWAY ALL MY TROUBLES, PAINS AND SORROWS. I WONDER WHY GOD HAS CHOSEN ME AND MY FAMILY TO SUFFER AND MOST IMPORTANTLY MY FATHER. I WONDER WHAT JUSTIFICATION THERE IS – OR IF THERE IS ANY AT ALL. MY LIFE FEELS THAT IT HAS BEGUN TO FALL APART, AND SCHOOL FEELS SO UNIMPORTANT.

I KNEW I NEEDED TO GO TO SCHOOL.

I ALWAYS FELT HAPPIER AND BETTER AFTER I HAD GONE TO SCHOOL AND COMPLETED MY ACTIVITIES. MY MOM AND I ALWAYS ENDED UP IN HUGE FIGHTS WHEN I DIDN'T FULFILL MY RESPONSIBILITIES. BY GOING TO SCHOOL, YOU AVOID SO MANY PROBLEMS AND DO NOT KEEP GETTING FURTHER AND FURTHER BEHIND IN YOUR SCHOOL WORK. THE WORST PART OF THE DAY IS WHEN YOU HAVE TO PUSH AND FORCE YOURSELF OUT OF BED, BUT YOU MAY BEGIN TO FEEL BETTER AND BETTER SLOWLY AS YOU BECOME MORE ACTIVE THROUGH YOUR DAY. FORCING MYSELF TO GET THROUGH THE DAY, GO TO SCHOOL AND DO MY AFTER SCHOOL ACTIVITIES HAS SERIOUSLY HELPED ME. THIS BENEFITED MY ENTIRE FAMILY BY NOT CAUSING THE ANGER, TURMOIL, AND FIGHTING BETWEEN ME AND MY MOM. FOR ME, SCHOOL WAS THE LAST THING OR PLACE I WANTED TO FACE AFTER LOSING MY DAD. BUT YOU HAVE TO FIND A ROUTINE AGAIN OR ELSE YOU MAY NEVER FIND ORDER IN YOUR LIFE AGAIN AND THE DARK CLOUD OVER YOU WILL CONTINUE TO GROW AND SPREAD TO EVERY ASPECT OF YOUR LIFE. LIVE TO MAKE YOUR PARENT EITHER SICK OR DECEASED PROUD.
THEY'RE WATCHING NO MATTER WHERE THEY ARE.

HAYDEN, AGE 16

A FRIEND IS ONE WHO WALKS IN WHEN THE REST OF THE WORLD WALKS OUT.

ANONYMOUS

When you are walking along in your life, thinking everything is great, and then, BAM, the word cancer intrudes, there are a lot of issues that run through your mind. Death. Loss. Confusion. Fear. The first things you think of don't usually include school, but that's a domineering factor in how a person deals with the c-word.

My childhood and schooling was pretty normal until my junior year, when my mom was diagnosed with breast cancer and I realized I couldn't function the same way at school. As hard as I tried, I couldn't make myself be happy. I trudge through my halls and classes unsmilingly and my grades slipped, all because the word "cancer" was tattooed across my mind's eye.
Just the thought of my mom alone wasn't the only thing I had to deal with at home my mom was actually physically suffering. Soon after she was diagnosed, she went in for treatment and surgery. I can clearly remember that day when she came home from the hospital. She was weak and in pain, and all I could do was put her to bed and try and take care of her the best I could.

I've never wanted to switch places with someone more in my life.

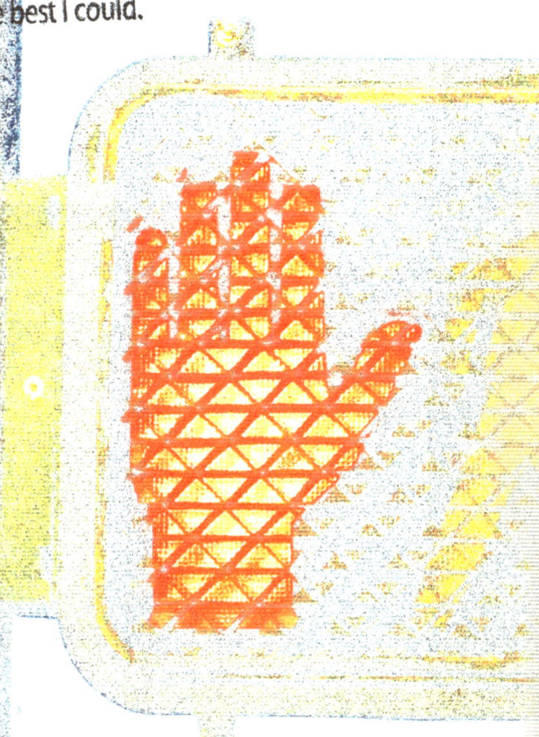

This stage in my life was like a vicious cycle – my mom's condition made it harder to be myself at school, and the fact that school sucked made it harder to deal with my mom. Although I wish this story had a phenomenally inspiring point that turned it all around, it really doesn't. My mom went into remission, and I was able to pick up the pieces and be Lydia again. I think to be able to dig myself out of my rut I had to realize that being depressed all of the time wouldn't make my mom get better, so eventually the state of my mom's health reflected my attitude: on good terms, but never quite the same as it had been before, and never would be again.

Lydia, age 18

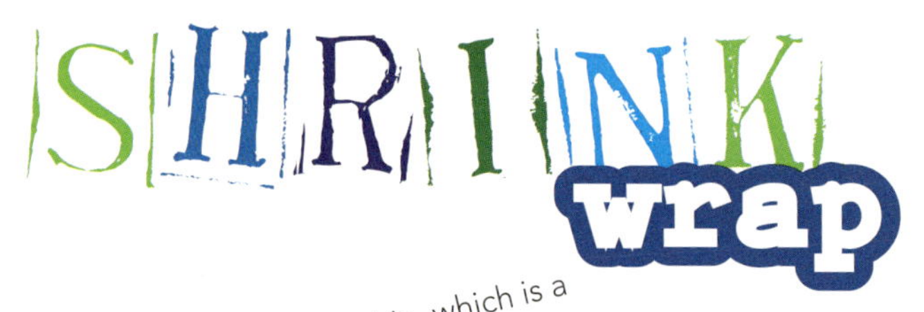

Avoiding school can turn into School Phobia, which is a form of anxiety. The problem with not going to school is this: The more you don't go, the more you don't go. And the more you don't go, the more your problems grow. You substitute immediate relief of the problem, which is the anxiety of going to school, with a much bigger problem of missing too much school, not doing your work and having your grades drop.

Often when you return to school after a day or two, your anxiety may even be increased because you have diverted from your usual routine. Routine helps keep anxiety under control. Facing issues or situations that may make you feel anxious also helps keep anxiety under control. The more you avoid anxiety producing situations, the more the anxiety grows.

- Lynnette

"The worst thing I hated the most was seeing my mom in pain. It hurts me so bad. Whenever my mom gets touched with a little bit of pressure there's a bruise almost instantly. There is almost no way to prevent it except for me to just stay away... but I can't. My mom's skin is very thin from the Decadron2 (A STEROID). My mom's skin rips almost instantly and then she's also taking blood thinners for her blood clots and whenever she gets a cut, blood just sprays everywhere and I have to put pressure on it until the doctors come to our house to tape it up. Her skin is so thin, she can't have stitches."

" My Mom also had radiation to her brain because the cancer spread there. Now she doesn't have any hair and she has to wear a wig to make her feel better. Since the cancer is in her brain, she cannot hear too well and she is very forgetful. It hurts me to see her say something 5 minutes ago and forget it and not even know what happened during that time. Another thing..my mom gets cramps from walking and so at night I go into her room whenever she needs me to rub away the cramps. The cramps are so huge that she screams and cries and the I start crying because I can't get them gone and it takes at least half an hour and then she gets another cramp in her next leg and then in her toes and sometimes I have to be rub- bing in 3 places at the same time and that's so hard for me because I get tired, but finally they go away and her legs are all purple from the cramps and she's tired."

Nick

16 years old

COOKING FOR MY MOM

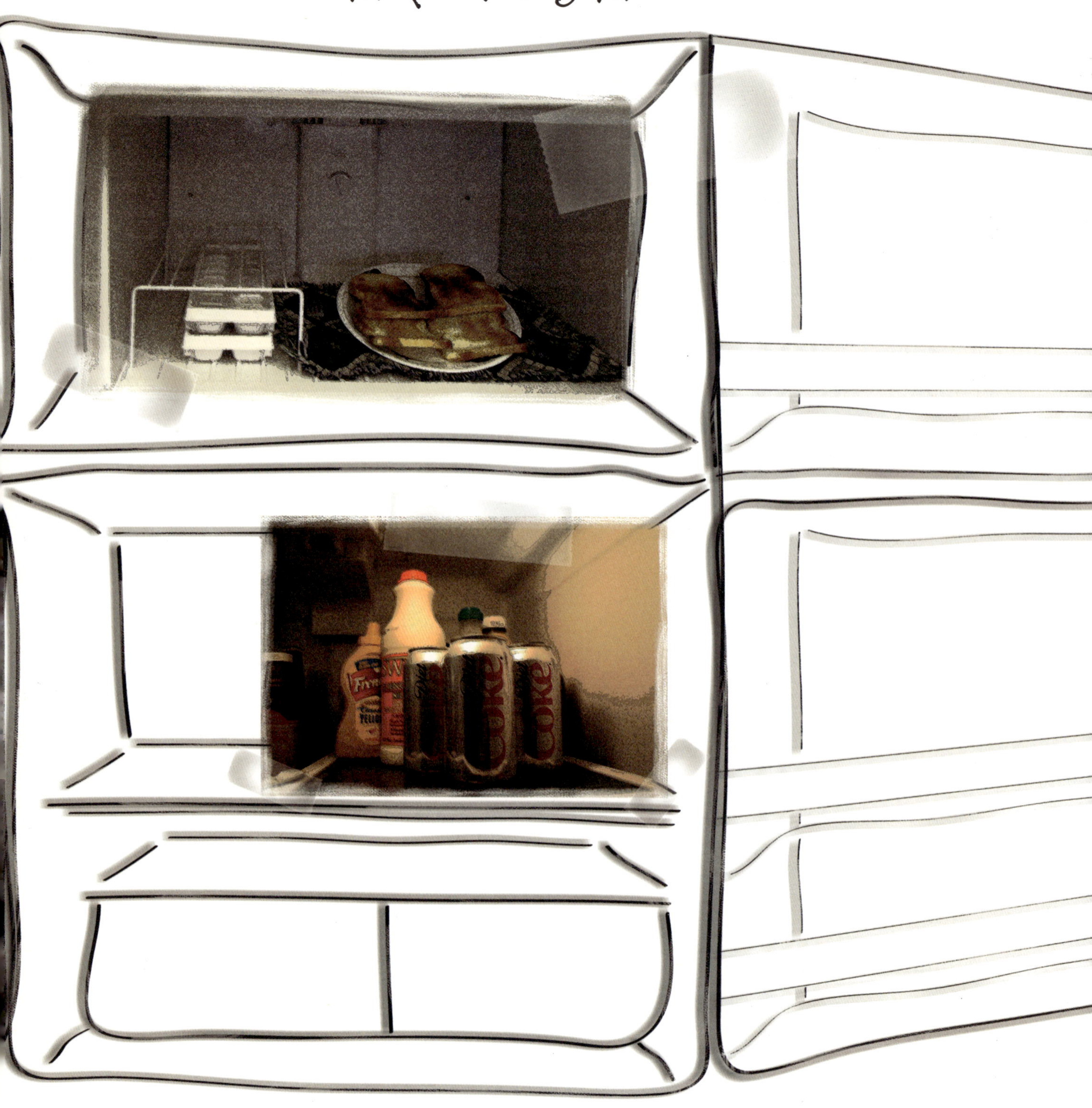

by Wynne, 16 years old

There's mashed potatoes made of flakes on the bottom shelf. They're beautiful sort of, she can always eat those. She's got nothing but she's still got something she can eat, more than I can say right now. The lights above the kitchen table aren't on, and I can see my reflection in the window above it. Cereal? No, that's a snack. I don't want to have to use the oven. Or the microwave. **Microwaves don't like tin foil.** Sixth graders aren't good cooks. I pull a bag of bread and untwist the red twisty tie. I take 2 slices of bread, which is soft and feels sort of wet. Back to the cupboard. Marmalade, I'm not in London. Nutella, three months old. Peanut butter, maybe. Refrigerator. Bologna with crispy edges, mayonnaise, Dijon mustard. Between both of my pantries. We got London and France, but still no meals. I shut the fridge door and listen for noise from the upstairs. There is none and I'm not sure if that's a good thing. Peanut butter and bread. Wait a second. Candy.

Mom's not awake. And I am. Chocolate's good on everything, reds and blues and green and browns, grab the other slice of bread and smashit! Put my creation on a plate. I listen again, and this time the silence beckons me like a whimpering puppy, I climb the stairs. The room is lit with a low lamp, and both of her legs are propped up against the wall. It's a yoga pose, the Supported Shoulder stand. She says it's the only comfortable position she's made a red mark on the white wall where her afghan has done 300 shoulder stands. Her skin its olive shade is thin, and her eyes are shut. I lie on the bed, it sags and I lean over to her. "Hey mom."

She opens her eyes and turns to me. "Hi."

"Do you want me to bring you anything?"

She smiles.

"Applesauce? Diet coke?"

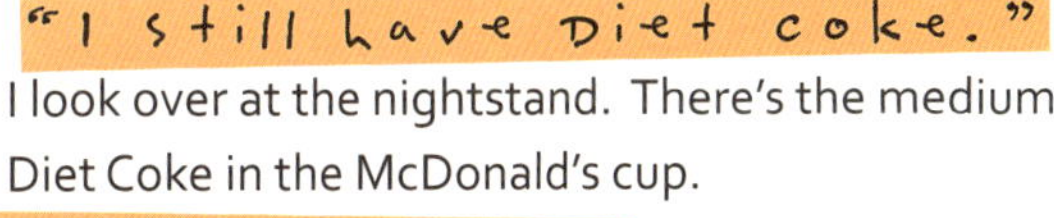

"I still have Diet coke."

I look over at the nightstand. There's the medium Diet Coke in the McDonald's cup.

"Thank you." She says.

"I made myself a sandwich." I say, not wanting to leave. Her eyes are shining at me. She's sorry, I can tell. She hates this, so how do her eyes still glisten? She looks like she's trying and she's still lying down. "Okay." I kiss her on the cheek. Her skin is cool, not cold. She smiles at me as I turn and climb off the bed. I look back at her and grin. As I walk down the stairs I feel as though I could run in two directions. Downstairs to my sandwich to the sanctuary of the television? To her room to lay down next to her and be. Which me will win? The one who aches for normalcy? The one who wants to comfort? The sandwich wins. The sandwich wins. Peanut butter is easier to understand. My dinner where I let it I turn on the TV and flip the channels. I don't turn on any of the lights. Not because I like the dark. Has anyone ever noticed we use too much light? The TV glows, do I need it to be illuminated more? The sandwich is thick, I won't be hungry. The sitcom blares.

Suddenly I get up, swing open the cupboards. A small dish is mine, I put it on the counter and get the applesauce from the fridge. Dish some up. Take it upstairs, I pause before I go in. I don't bother to wake her up, but my presence makes her open her eyes. She's glistening at me again. Makes me upset, I didn't bring 100 applesauces. But she seems happy with one. I set it on the nightstand.

"Just in case," I tell her.

Smiling. "Thanks I'll eat it in a little bit."

We both know she won't. But as I sit next to her on the bed, we both know that's not why I brought it.

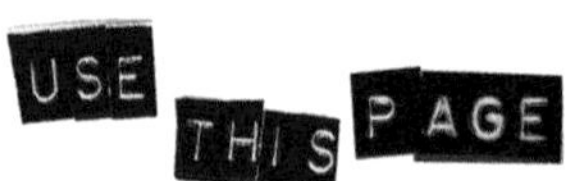
USE THIS PAGE

how do you see the world now?

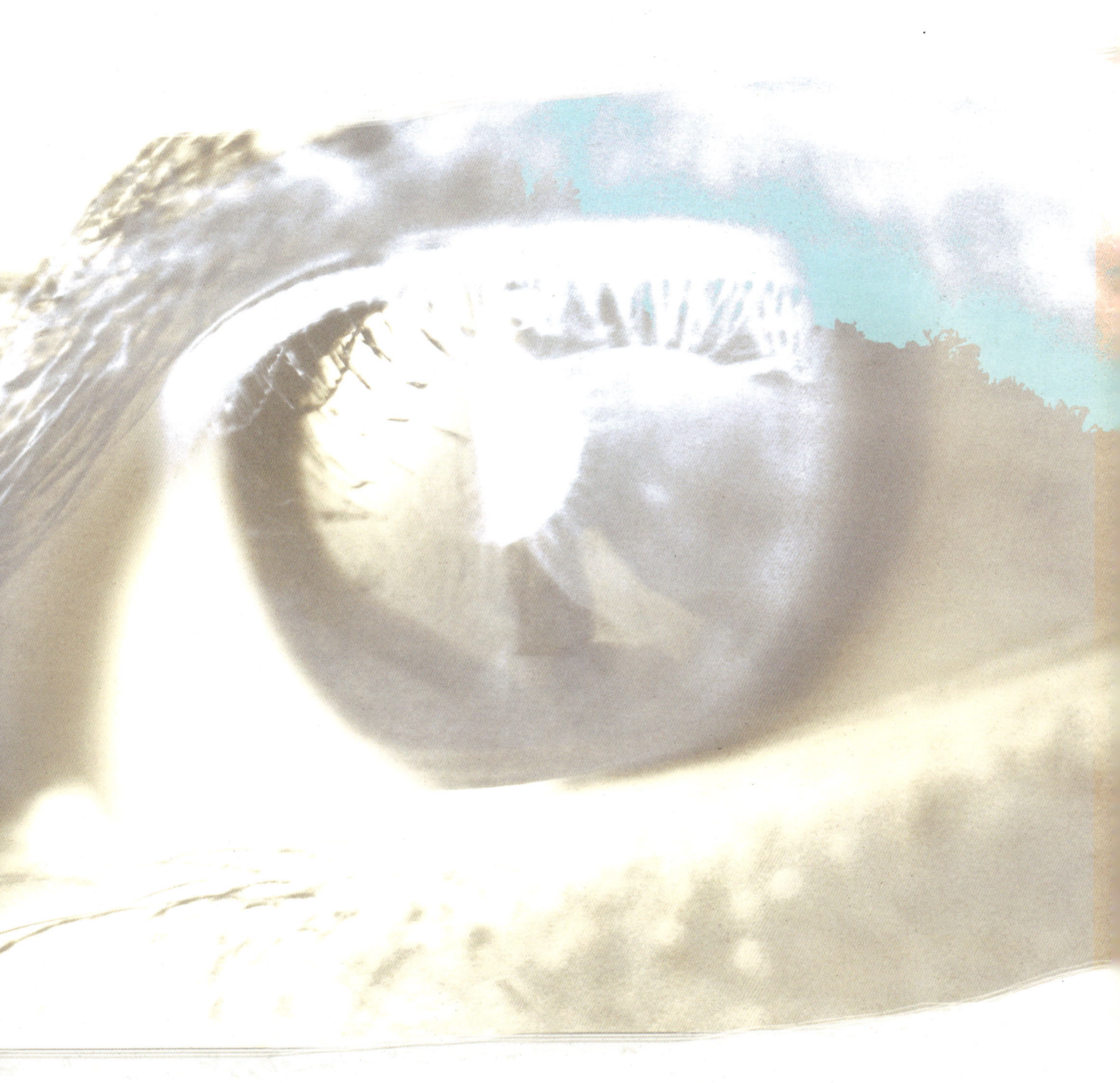

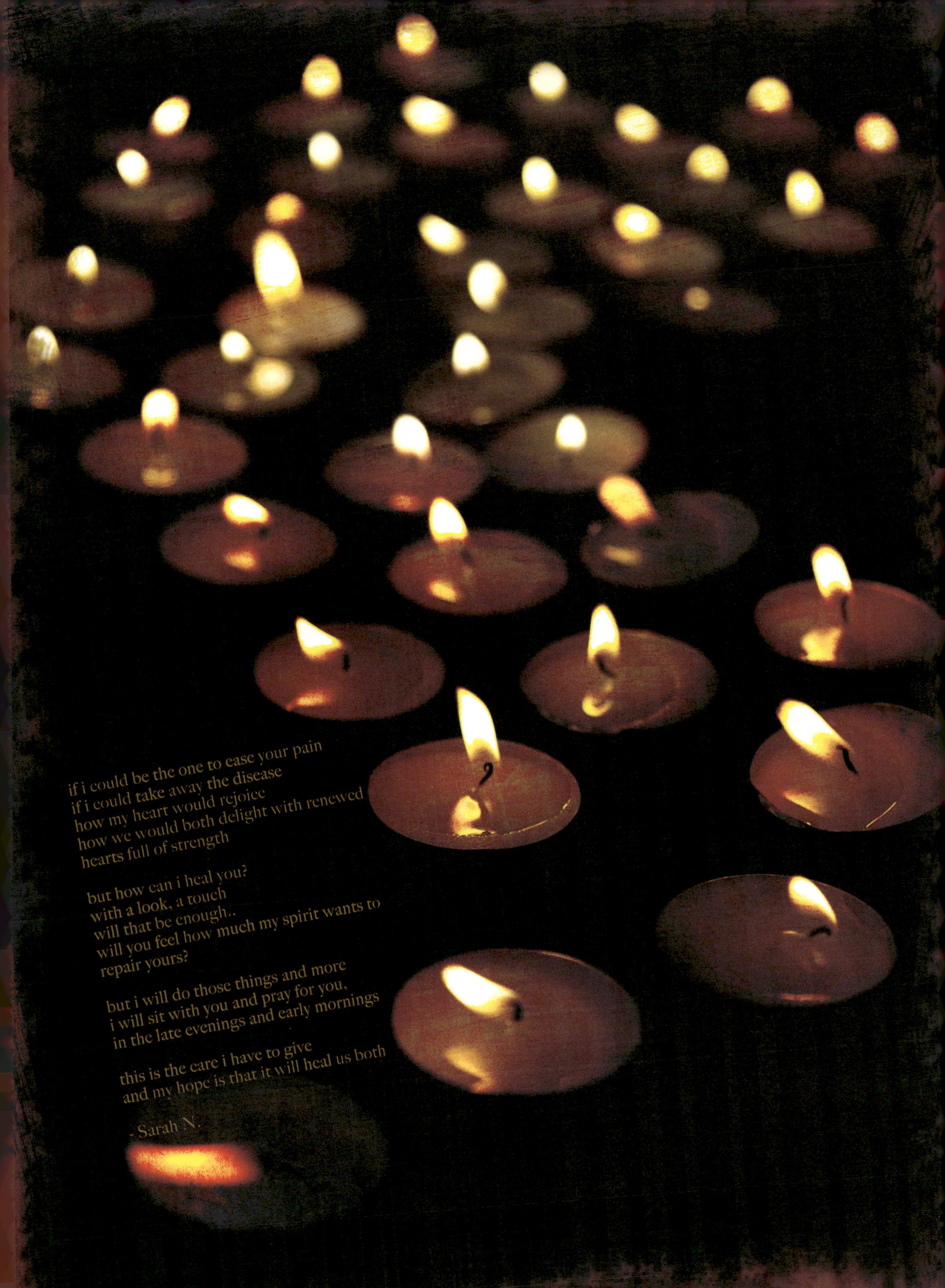
if i could be the one to ease your pain
if i could take away the disease
how my heart would rejoice
how we would both delight with renewed
hearts full of strength

but how can i heal you?
with a look, a touch
will that be enough..
will you feel how much my spirit wants to
repair yours?

but i will do those things and more
i will sit with you and pray for you,
in the late evenings and early mornings

this is the care i have to give
and my hope is that it will heal us both

- Sarah N.

I have been told by many teens that one of the most difficult aspects of dealing with a parent's cancer treatment is when they are put in the role of being the caregiver. It can't get more annoying than having to drive your younger sibling to soccer practice or help make dinner or even drive your parent to their doctor's appointments when you have plans with friends or just want to get out of the house.

SHRINK wrap

You do have the choice of either resenting the requests or having a good attitude about helping.

When you approach this situation in a positive helpful way, you just might start to feel a sense of pride. You might also find that your relationships with their siblings will become closer.

Try to remember, no one has chosen this situation, no one wants to have to burden you. It just is what it is, so everyone has to just make the best of it. Helping out the family with a "good" attitude takes a huge burden off of your parents; having a "bad" attitude about it only adds to the burden.

- Lynnette

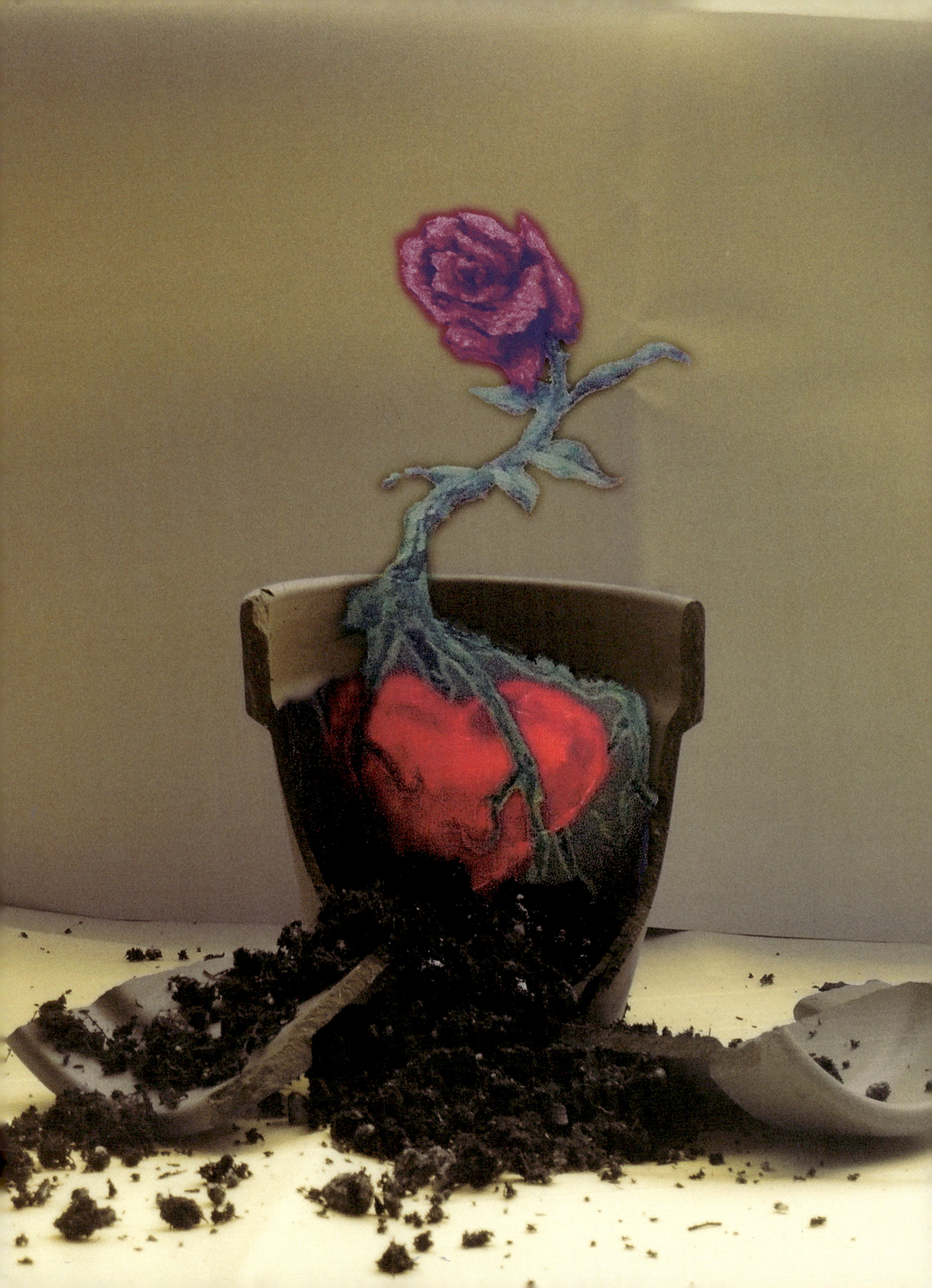

For the last 9 years I have felt a "hole" in me.

I can even tell you where it is. It is right below my sternum and a bit to the left. It's not a hole made by a gun shot wound or surgery or from a death defying stunt gone wrong; it's a hole in me that is all my loneliness, alienation and bitterness. These emotions act as a parasite would or a corrosive acid, eating away at the wall of the hole making it a larger chasm, making me painfully aware of my loneliness and my separateness from others.

I became aware of this hole after the death of my mother, she died when I was nine years old of breast cancer. As I got older I realized the consequences of this event more and more, simultaneously becoming aware of this hole. As my awareness of its existence grew, I consciously began to recognize these emotions and the greater pain I felt from them. I felt that the loss of my mother made me incomplete, such that I would miss out on crucial elements that I would otherwise experience as a child and a teenager. I felt that I would miss out on being the recipient of love and care, that others would receive and I would not. Perhaps the hole was caused by my mother's death, certainly the experience affected me in a profound way. I think that event caused the hole, and each passing worry, frustration, fear and bitter taste in my mouth widened the hole a bit further. Once you experience grief, at a young age, you are forced to grow up. There is no going back after this experience. For me, the effects of experiencing grief was this feeling of emptiness, this "hole " .

I write this from the vantage point of a young man who has just finished his first year of college and from this point I see that the culmination point of the loneliness and anxiety was in October of my freshman year of college. It was at this point in time which I tried to fill this hole. My attempts, however only served to patch it. I used distractions both consciously and unconsciously to fill the hole. However, like a pit poorly filled with dirt, it is always evident to the passing viewer that there once was a hole there and a hideous scar is left on the ground.

The hole is primarily a symbol for feeling alone, left to your own devices, and the pain that is derived from that. Bitterness, anger, and sadness are also associated with the hole, and for me, they can make the hole feel larger and more powerful. However, I recognize that these are not only symptoms of a person whose parent has been lost to a tumor; these are also feelings present in every adolescent, and thus I cannot determine infallibly that the death of a parent is the cause of them. Thus the hole is symbol of everyone's loneliness, of everyone's desire to connect with others, also showing the imperfection of human beings and revealing aspects of the human condition. And invariably the hole becomes a symbol of my humanity as well. So my point is not that only teenagers in a similar situation to my own go through this, my point is that the loss of a parent has a profound and perhaps amplifying effect on such feelings and the hole overall.

- - - - >

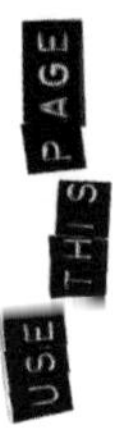

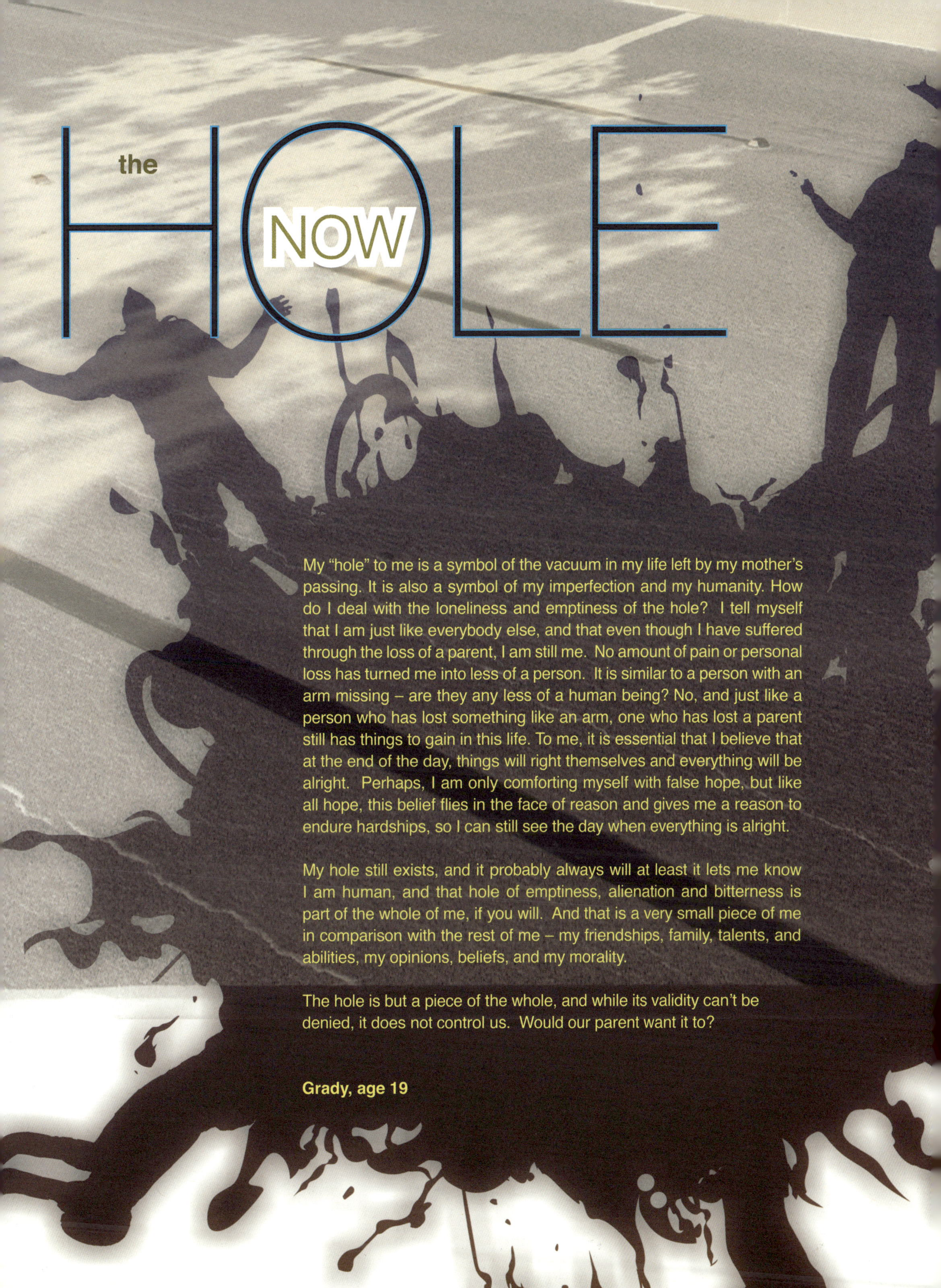

the HOLE NOW

My "hole" to me is a symbol of the vacuum in my life left by my mother's passing. It is also a symbol of my imperfection and my humanity. How do I deal with the loneliness and emptiness of the hole? I tell myself that I am just like everybody else, and that even though I have suffered through the loss of a parent, I am still me. No amount of pain or personal loss has turned me into less of a person. It is similar to a person with an arm missing – are they any less of a human being? No, and just like a person who has lost something like an arm, one who has lost a parent still has things to gain in this life. To me, it is essential that I believe that at the end of the day, things will right themselves and everything will be alright. Perhaps, I am only comforting myself with false hope, but like all hope, this belief flies in the face of reason and gives me a reason to endure hardships, so I can still see the day when everything is alright.

My hole still exists, and it probably always will at least it lets me know I am human, and that hole of emptiness, alienation and bitterness is part of the whole of me, if you will. And that is a very small piece of me in comparison with the rest of me – my friendships, family, talents, and abilities, my opinions, beliefs, and my morality.

The hole is but a piece of the whole, and while its validity can't be denied, it does not control us. Would our parent want it to?

Grady, age 19

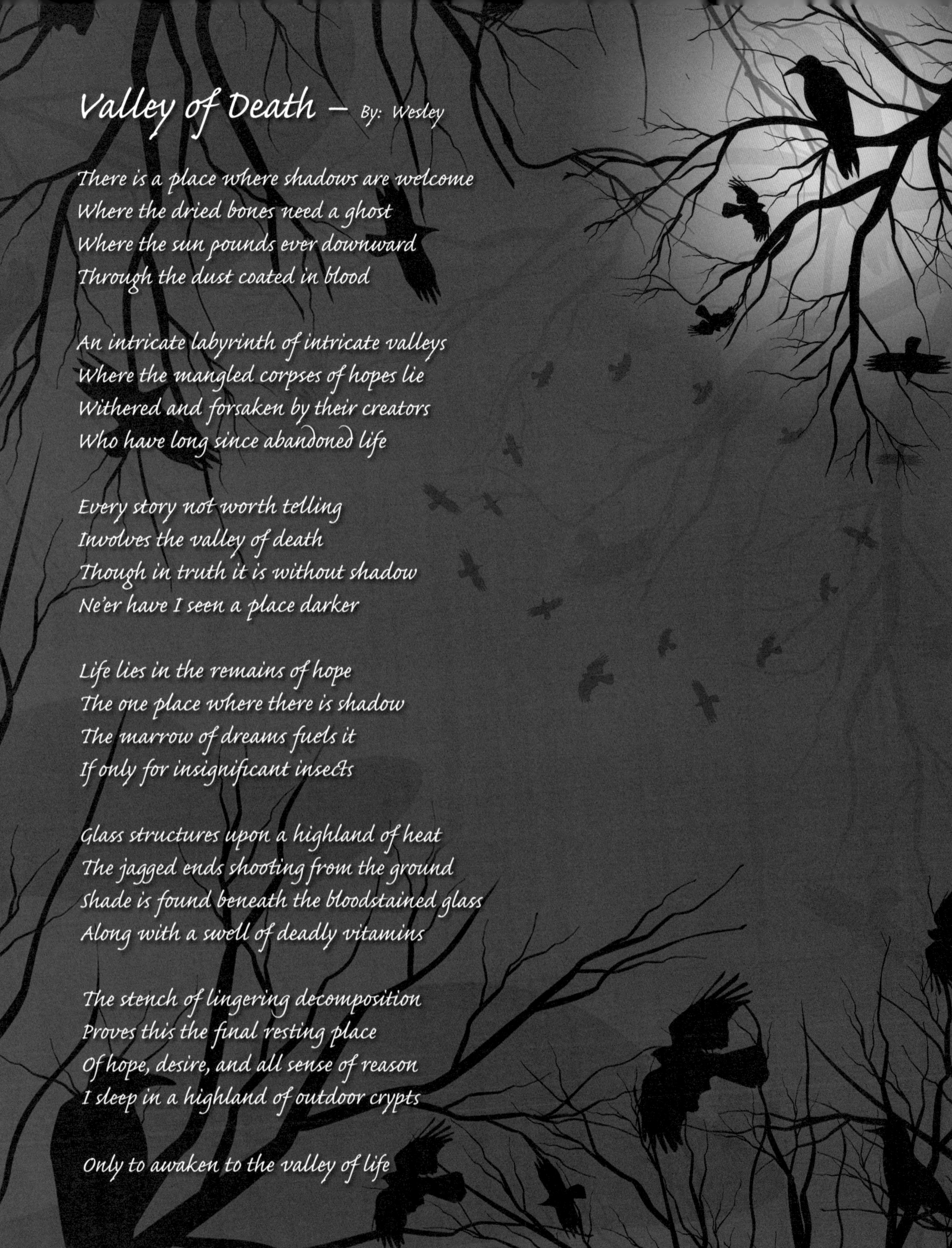

Valley of Death – By: Wesley

There is a place where shadows are welcome
Where the dried bones need a ghost
Where the sun pounds ever downward
Through the dust coated in blood

An intricate labyrinth of intricate valleys
Where the mangled corpses of hopes lie
Withered and forsaken by their creators
Who have long since abandoned life

Every story not worth telling
Involves the valley of death
Though in truth it is without shadow
Ne'er have I seen a place darker

Life lies in the remains of hope
The one place where there is shadow
The marrow of dreams fuels it
If only for insignificant insects

Glass structures upon a highland of heat
The jagged ends shooting from the ground
Shade is found beneath the bloodstained glass
Along with a swell of deadly vitamins

The stench of lingering decomposition
Proves this the final resting place
Of hope, desire, and all sense of reason
I sleep in a highland of outdoor crypts

Only to awaken to the valley of life

Living without a Mom – Wynne 16 yrs

HAVE YOU EVER BOUGHT TAMPONS WITH YOUR DAD?
HE'S ACTUALLY LOOKING AT THE BRANDS. OH GOD, PLEASE STOP. WHAT IS HE DOING?
IS HE PICKING ONE UP? "HOW ABOUT THESE?" OH MY GOD – MAKE IT STOP.
HOW MANY TIMES HAVE I SAID THAT LATELY? AND NOT JUST ABOUT THE GENERIC BOX OF
TAMPONS, MY DAD IS HOLDING RIGHT NOW IN PUBLIC. IF I WISH MY LIFE WEREN'T MINE ONE
MORE TIME I THINK I MIGHT BE SICK.. WHY CAN'T I JUST OWN WHAT'S HAPPENING TO ME?
WHY CAN'T I RESPECT DAD FOR TRYING? HE'S HERE IS HE NOT? HE'S HOLDING THE WRONG
BRAND BUT HE'S STILL HOLDING SOMETHING. WHY ISN'T HE HOLDING ME? I WISH HE WOULD.
MAYBE NOT IN THE FEMININE HYGIENE AISLE, BUT THAT'S SOMETHING SHE WOULD DO THAT
HE DOESN'T. THERE'S A LOT OF THINGS SHE DID, HE DOESN'T. HOLD ME, CALL ME AFTER WORK,
MAKE ME POTPIES, CALL ME A NICKNAME THAT WAS JUST MINE, DO EMBARRASSING STUFF LIKE
THIS FOR ME. I GRAB THE BOX FROM HIM, PUT IT BACK AND GET THE RIGHT ONE.
PUSH THE CART FORWARD, PRAY THAT HE'S FOLLOWING ME. HE USUALLY IS.

BEING 17 AND A GIRL AND ONLY HAVING A DAD IS LIKE THIS. MY DAD DIDN'T
PULL A SHOT GUN ON THE LAST BOYFRIEND I HAD. HE DID SOMETHING WORSE.
HE MADE A 17 YEAR OLD BOY PROVE HIS LOYALTY.
DOESN'T HE KNOW THAT FORCING ANYONE TO PROVE THEIR LOYALTY IS RISKY?
ESPECIALLY A HORMONAL LOYALIST.
WHY CAN'T HE JUST TRUST?
WHY DOES HE HAVE TO WALK SLOWLY OUT OF THIS AISLE RIGHT NOW?
WHY DOES HE HAVE TO BE DIFFERENT THAN MOM? WHY ISN'T HE A GIRL?
MOM WOULD'VE LOVED MY LAST BOYFRIEND.... I THINK.
SHE WOULD BUY TAMPONS HERSELF,
AND SHE WOULDN'T MAKE ME PROVE ANYTHING.

I WATCH MY GIRLFRIEND ANSWER HER CELL PHONE ON OUR LUNCH BREAK.
SHE ROLLS HER EYES TO DANGEROUS ATTITUDES INSIDE HER SKULL. "IT'S MY MOM."
SHE OPENS THE PHONE AND SPITS, "WHAT?" I REALIZE THEN THAT I WOULD'VE ANSWERED
THE PHONE EXACTLY THE SAME IF IT WERE MY DAD. I AM IT, I AM A YOUNG WOMAN.
I AM SMART, AND BEAUTIFUL, AND WELL SPOKEN, OUT GOING, CONFUSED, PASSIONATE, LOUD.
I AM ALL OF THOSE THINGS; I HAVE BECOME THOSE THINGS WITH
AND WITHOUT MY MOM.

I REALIZE THEN THE MAN IN FRONT OF ME IN A WORKOUT
SWEATSHIRT, JEANS AND UTILITY SNEAKERS HOLDING THE GENERIC BOX
OF TAMPONS HAS STRUGGLED WITH ME BEING THOSE THINGS.
AND LOVED ME STILL.
HOW DID MOM KNOW HE'D DO THAT AND I DIDN'T?
MOMS' JUST KNOW EVERYTHING I GUESS!!

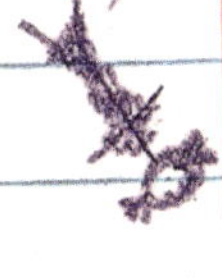

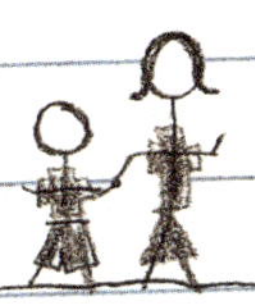
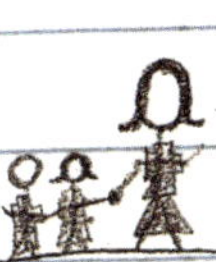
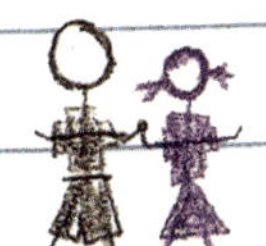
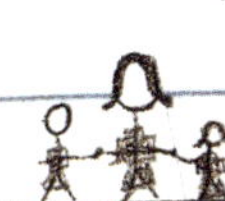
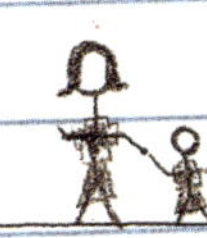

WHEN DAD DIED

The phone rang around nine o'clock and Dr. John Demman was on the other end asking for Mom. I told him Mom was at work and asked him how Dad was since I had not seen him since yesterday. He said that Dad was semi-comatose, and he was not sure how long it would be. I freaked out, hung up the phone and ran into my brother's room, **I WAS SCREAMING AND SOBBING, TELLING HIM TO GET UP AND DRIVE ME TO SEE DAD.** We headed to the hospital as fast as we could get there. I was scared, and I knew deep down I had to tell him the one thing that I did not want to say. I sat in the hospital room, holding my Dad's hand and **TOLD HIM THAT I LOVED HIM FOREVER AND THAT I WOULD BE OKAY IF HE WAS READY TO DIE.** I knew from going to Kids Konnected support groups that it was very important to say, "good-bye."

Later that day, my Dad died, alone in his hospital room.

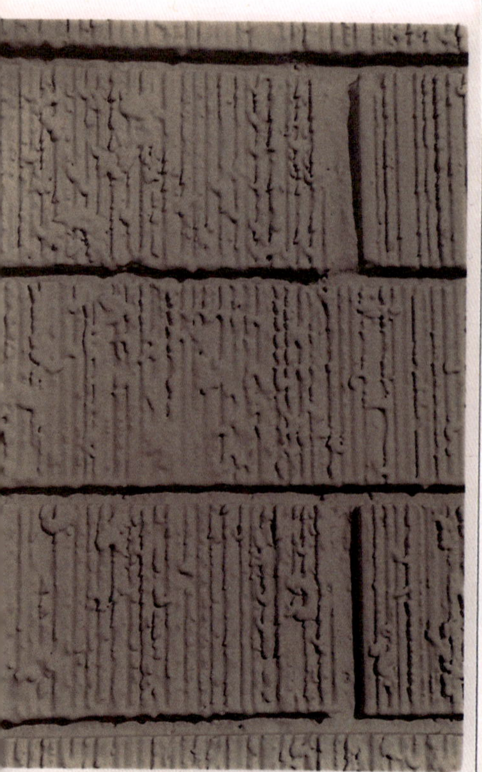

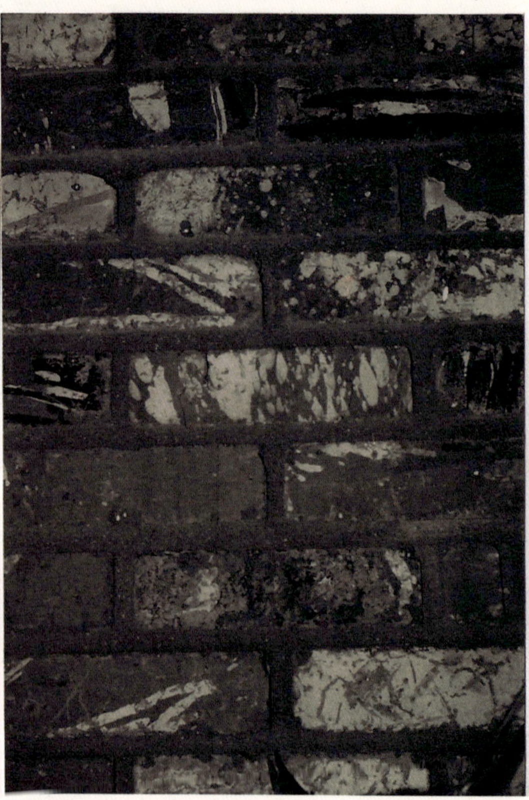

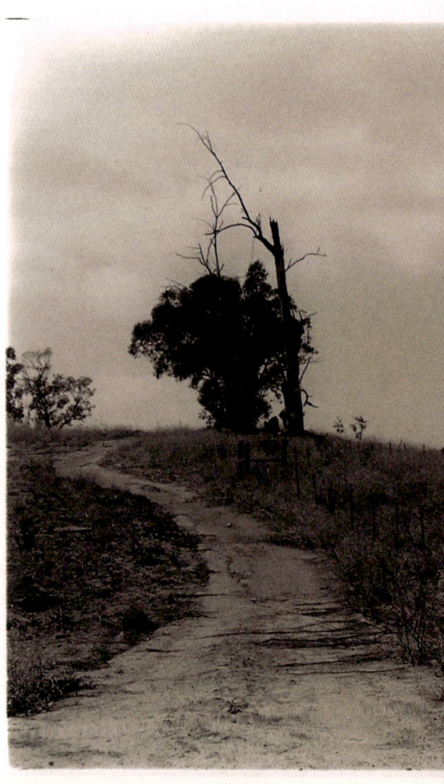

Once we were seated in the front now facing the casket, that was when I realized that he was really gone. The funeral was nice considering it was a funeral. As we were walking out of the chapel to proceed to the gravesite, I saw Robyn Holtz, from Kids Konnected. Her son started Kids Konnected. She had never met my Dad, had only known me for a few months, but was there to support me. We made our way to the gravesite and the hardest thing for me was to see them lowering the casket into the ground, because once again it made everything that was happening real, and that **THE REALITY OF IT ALL WAS THAT HE WAS GONE FOREVER AND MY LIFE WAS NOW GOING TO BE DIFFERENT FOREVER.**

Once I went back to school, I didn't want to be there with everyone saying how sorry they were, and to let them know if I needed anything to just ask. **YES I DID NEED SOMETHING, AND THAT WAS TO HAVE EVERYONE LEAVE ME THE HELL ALONE.** Sarah, age 18

Alright, I am gonna try to say this without sounding too much like a therapist. So how do you deal with the death/diagnosis of a parent? Where do you turn? What do you do with the questions and uncertainty of the situation? There are many ways to deal with it — smoke a little pot, drink a bit, hang out with friends, write in a journal, cut your arm, the point is there is a sea of distraction to get lost in. And in the rush of the situation and pain, it is easy to choose an option that can harm yourself or another person. For me the best definition of a healthy way of dealing with it, is an outlet that allows me to be myself and express myself constructively. It doesn't change me or bind me. It took me a while to find an outlet that actually worked for me in a positive way.

My first reaction to a bad situation is to get angry. Very angry. Because when I am angry, I feel powerful enough to handle anything, to change the unchangeable, even though I know that is not actually possible. But it doesn't matter if it's actually possible, because it feels so good and in that angry, adrenaline filled moment, you feel like you can take on factors out of your control and bend them to your will. But in truth, there are still things out of your control, and began to lash out at my family and friends. **The worst part was that I didn't care; I loved feeling angry, and wanted to stay that way.** Feeling control was my way of avoiding feeling helpless in a situation out of my control.

Then music came into my life. I began to listen to the music of my parents' generation, and rather than feel angry and hit something, I could listen to Jimi Hendrix playing Voodoo Child. It was like hearing my angst and troubles expressed in a way that made me feel just as good as when I was angry. Rather than feel in control because of an adrenaline rush, I felt content. My dad also got me my first guitar my freshman year of high school. Somehow playing music felt better than heckling my siblings to make them feel as miserable as I was.

Perhaps unconsciously, I wanted people to identity with me. Anger became my way of letting people know I was miserable, and I wanted them to know exactly how I felt. I made them miserable, so I could have someone to share my misery with.

But in the raw power of music, of strings bending on a guitar or notes hammered out on a piano, I could feel the emotions, the highs and lows, which paralleled and echoed my own. I began to identify with the feeling of the music, and I began to express myself through it. Now there are calluses on my fingertips, instead of bruises on my knuckles.

The point of that whole story is that there are better ways to deal with a loss than resorting to an addiction to anger, pot, or cutting yourself. Once you use one of those outlets you run the risk of using it as a crutch to prop yourself up. But when you play music, hang with a friend, or write or read a book, you are you, and you are creating something out of your sorrow, rather than allowing it to direct you.

Grady, age 18

Dealing with Feelings -

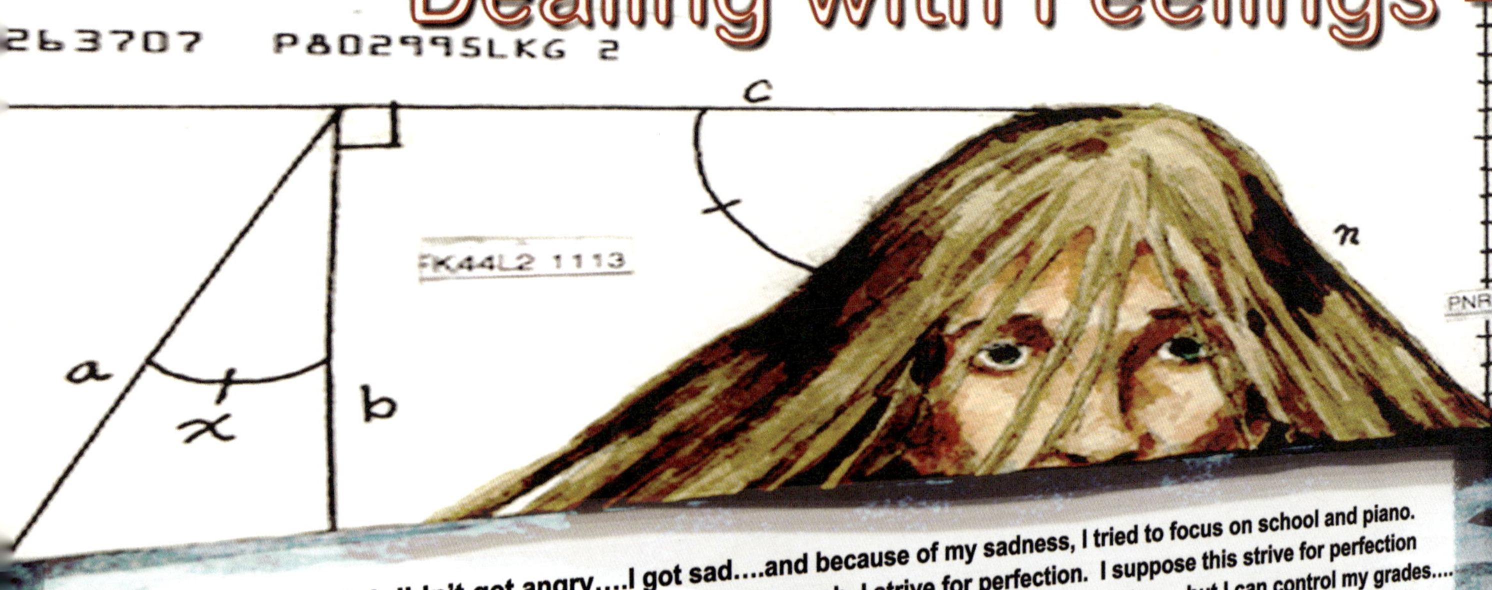

When my Dad died, I didn't get angry….I got sad….and because of my sadness, I tried to focus on school and piano. But the problem with my focusing is that I focus too much, I strive for perfection. I suppose this strive for perfection is a way for me to control "something" in my life. I mean, I can't control my father dying….but I can control my grades…. I think?? Everyone knows what it's like to cry so hard that you can't breathe. Everyone knows what it's like to be crushed with disappointment when you just can't get what you want. But not everyone knows what it's like to feel that kind of intense frustration and depression when you realize that you can't be perfect.

Everyone knows a few of us. We're the ones who fly into hysterics when we miss that one question or the test when everyone else is happy to get a B, we're the ones who drive you insane with our nit-picky obsession to be flawless. There's a word for us crazy circus folk: perfectionists. You might think us lucky to have such intense drive and motivation, the kind of thing that makes us excel in school and seemingly, in everything we do. Think again. Beneath the cool and collected façade, that burning desire to be perfect just leaves us wallowing in a puddle of our own shortcomings. My own problems with perfectionism started in sixth grade when school started getting more competitive. I had always excelled in school prior to junior high, so why shouldn't I be the best in my grade now? Well, I got my wish, school was easy for me, but I worked hard anyway so I could be that much better.
I was perfect.
I was happy.

By the time I got to eighth grade, however, I started to realize that I had gotten carried away with perfection. I remember beating myself up for days after I discovered that I hadn't earned every single point in English, even though I had gotten well over a hundred percent in that class. At the time, I thought that what I was doing was normal, even healthy,because it caused me to try harder, resulting in higher grades and more academic success. In high school, things got even harder. Because of the push I had given myself in middle school, I was taking accelerated classes in which I thought I could easily succeed. For the most part, I was right. Where I did not succeed, however, was in Honors Algebra II. I did well until March, when all the pressure I had put on myself to be the perfect student and person finally crushed me. For the first time, I failed a test. I spent all of lunch crying in a bathroom that day, and when I came home I bawled for hours in my room. It was then that I realized that I couldn't be perfect, and that I would only be unhappy if I pursued perfection. I earned my first B in a class that semester and while at the time it seemed as if the world could swallow me up and I wouldn't live, I learned a very valuable lesson from the experience.

I am now in tenth grade. I am still a perfectionist, but I have worked to accept myself more for who I am, not what I have accomplished. I currently have a B in Honors Chemistry and that is just fine with me, because I have the satisfaction of knowing that I tried my best. No one can be perfect at everything. Perfection in itself is an imperfection so trying to be flawless will just eat away at you from the inside, until you have sacrificed everything important to you. I am worthwhile, talented, intelligent and secure with my character and personality. This is all I need to be.

Allison, 15 years old

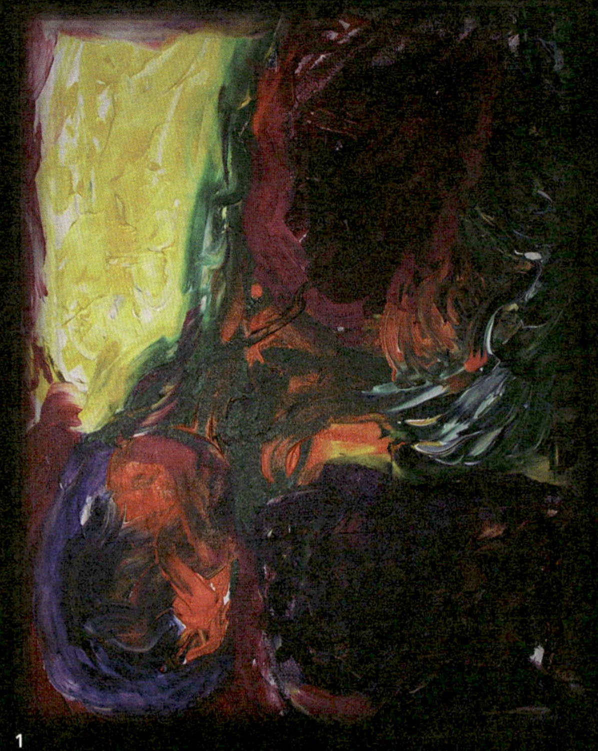

1

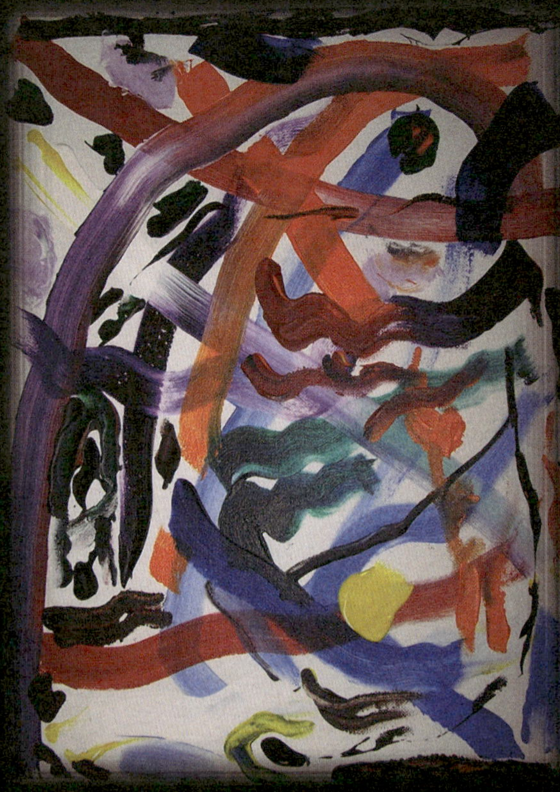

2

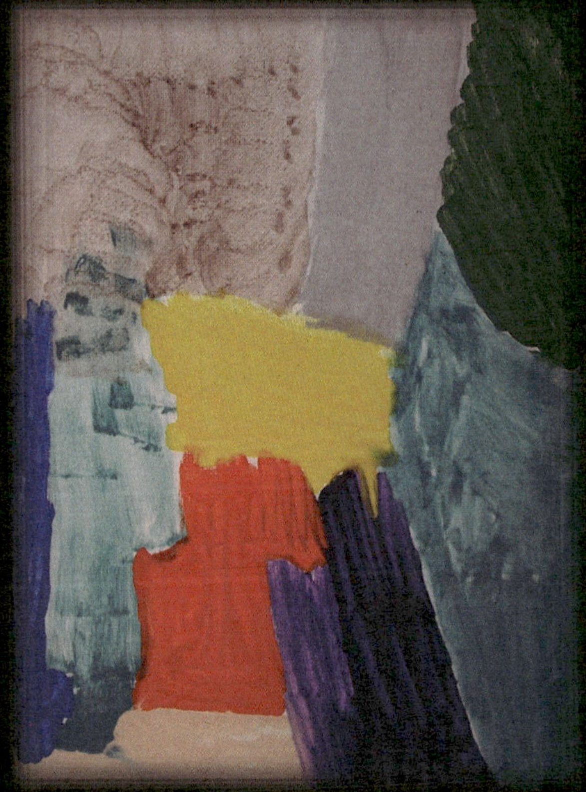

3

this page
1. losing my dad to cancer
2. a look inside my heart
3. fear

opposite page
4. all about me
5. anger

Jennifer's paintings

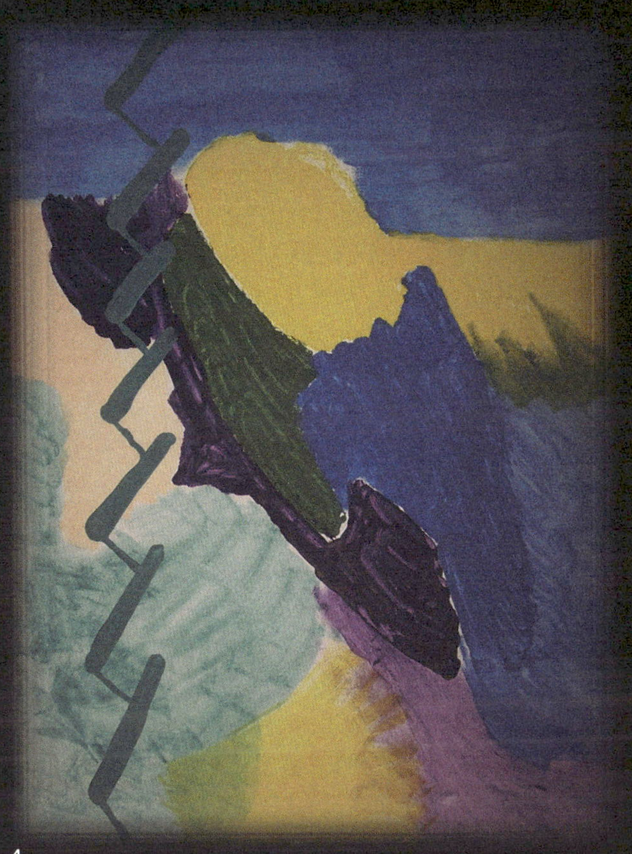

4

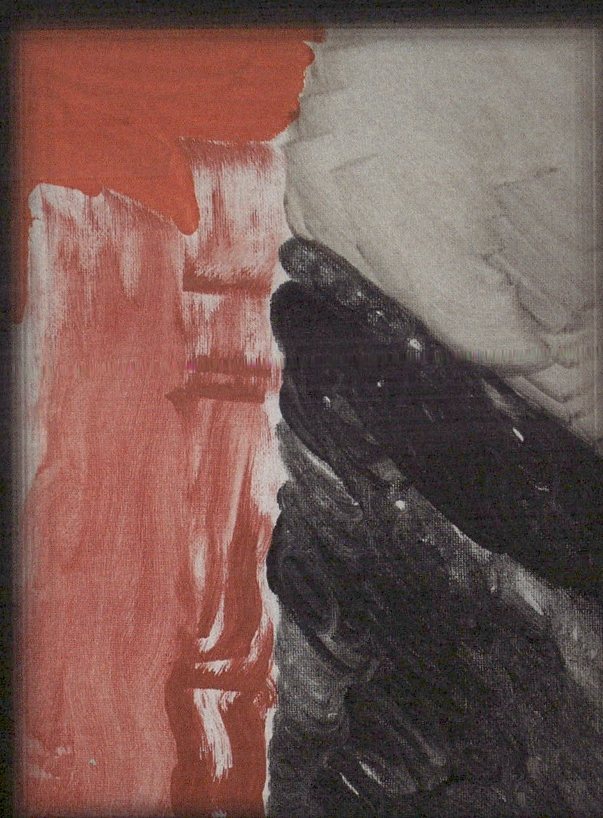

5

Jennifer's Story

We used to travel a lot, so one summer we were going to travel in a motor home cross-country. We bought a brand new motor home from a dealership in Las Vegas. We were going to get the shower fixed because it was rattling and then it happened. I didn't know what was happening but my dad was shaking with his hands off the steering wheel and I couldn't wake him up. Later I found out that he was having a seizure. I saw a lady that was walking the same way that we were going. I tried to yell to her to get out of the way, but she obviously could not hear me through the motor home walls. The giant rear view mirror hit her in the back of the head and she fell over. Later I found out that the motor home rolled over her leg and broke it. I really didn't care because I didn't know what was happening to my dad and she only had a broken leg — that could be fixed. My mom was in front of us and he hit her as she was turning right. Our possessions that were packed into the rental car she was driving sprayed across the street. We went straight into a sign for an apartment complex and knocked over a giant palm tree. I hit my head on the panel that outlines the cab on impact while trying to get my dad to wake up. I could hardly get out because the door was stuck behind a stop sign. This guy dressed in army fatigue bent it back for me to get out. These kids that had come out from their apartment were laughing. LAUGHING!!! at my dad who was still seizing. I wanted to tell them to shut up but I was so deep in shock I don't remember if I did or not. The people from the motor home dealer came over and were able to shut off the gas — I would say luckily we were right next to the motor home dealer, but nothing from this experience can be described as lucky. The first ambulance went to help the lady and then they came to help my dad. I was really mad at them for doing that. He was hurt worse than she was. I was trying to pick our stuff up out of the street so that cars wouldn't run over it. I was hysterical. I could only think about our possessions getting ruined because I had no sense of what had happened to my dad. Then my mom told me to only pick up the important things and shove them back into the rental car because my dad was hurt and he needed us. The ambulance people had a hard time getting my dad out of the motor home because he was disoriented and thought they were trying to capture him. I rode in the front seat of one of the ambulances. My mom had gone in my dad's ambulance and the one that I was in didn't have anyone in the back. I wanted to know where my parents were, but the people took me to the

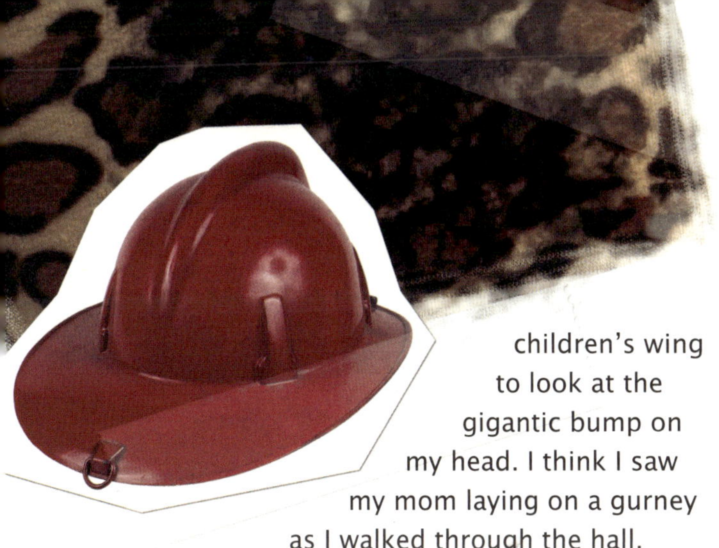

children's wing to look at the gigantic bump on my head. I think I saw my mom laying on a gurney as I walked through the hall. They gave me a cat — I think — Beanie Baby. I almost had a concussion. Then I went to see my mom who was laying in a bed with a giant neck brace on. She had got whiplash. I think she had seen my dad passing through the hall earlier even though I hadn't. Someone suggested that we go get a room at the hotel across the street where many of the patients' families stayed. We ate dinner at A&W even though I wasn't hungry. I was sick to my stomach with anxiety and fear. When we went back to the room, we turned on the tv and the news was broadcasting from the scene of the accident. That was crushing, to know that everywhere else in Las Vegas people were having fun gambling and playing arcade games and we were the topic of a news report. I don't think we saw my dad until the next day. I don't remember seeing him in the hospital. My mom and I had to do everything for ourselves. We went to the back of Target one night and took boxes that we could put our stuff in from the motor home and rental car. We also rented a U-Haul truck to put everything in. I remember we had to go to Office Depot to buy a lock so that people would not steal our stuff out of the truck. We went to the motor home dealership to get everything out of the motor home because it had been totaled. We also went to the car rental place to get everything out of the rental car. I was very sad because the firemen had sprayed a lot of our belongings with some kind of stuff so that the car wouldn't catch on fire. So much stuff was ruined. Our whole lives were in those vehicles and it was all ruined. I remember going to get our stuff out of the rental car and I saw a certificate that I had gotten and it was ripped and dirty and sitting on the ledge of the broken left back window. Also, my favorite purse backpack that my aunt had bought me for Christmas was ruined. It was a fuzzy cheetah print little backpack that I took everywhere. My mom said that we could replace our possessions but we could not replace my dad. One night in the hotel room, the son of the lady called and was angry that my dad had done this. I wanted to scream at him so much. I was so mad at him for thinking that my dad had any way to control himself from not having a seizure. We called my parent's friends and paid for them to fly to Las Vegas so that they could drive the U-Haul truck to our house because we had to fly home with my dad. I don't know exactly how long we were in Las Vegas — I think it was three or four days — but I wanted to get out of there. When we got home everything was different. My mom and dad went to doctor's appointments every day in Fountain Valley and at UCLA. I had to explain to my friends why I was home and not half way across the country. They were understanding, but didn't know how to react. I went into fifth grade that September. One day my parents had me come into their room and sit in bed with them. They told me that my dad has cancer and that he was sick. I was devastated. When I went to school the psychologist took me to her office and asked me what my parents had told me. I had blocked the fact that my dad had cancer so far out of my head that I had made myself forget. She told me that my dad had cancer and then I remembered that my parents had already told me. One day we were in health class and this girl that I hated because she was so annoying was reading an article and said the word seizure. I started crying. I got to go sit in the hall and I asked that my friend come out with me. I remember that someone gave me a booklet of papers stapled together for me to draw or write in. I drew Hope the bear that I had gotten from Kids Konnected so I think that I had just gotten the box. My friend said that I should cry more often to get us out of class. That was the most selfish comment I have ever heard and we were only ten. I didn't have to go to health again, but I sat out by myself. I wasn't going to let her benefit from my pain. I should have stopped being friends with her because from then on she only caused me pain and grief. But, I had no other friends to turn to so I stuck with her. Then there was a sub named Ms. Dugdale. I really liked her and she was very caring and kind. Mrs. Avzeradel was out having a baby. Then a new sub came because Ms. Dugdale had a family emergency.

I hated the new sub. She was fat and obnoxious. I don't remember much about being at home during those times. I know that we went on a trip up the coast that winter break. Then we got my dog on my birthday January 7. In the summer after fifth grade we went camping to Sequoia and Yosemite. We were only supposed to be gone for a week, but my dad loved being in nature so much. My mom thinks that he lived longer because we stayed in the mountains for so long. We had so much fun. It was like a last hurrah for us. We stayed there for almost the whole summer, but my dad got dehydrated and had to go to the hospital so then we went home. I stayed at my friend's house almost every day because my parents had to drive back and forth from UCLA and sometimes they stayed at my grandma's house. We had to get a hospital bed put in our house. At first a nurse came sometimes and then there was one all the time. I remember staying up until one in the morning several nights with my mom watching my dad. His mind and body began to deteriorate. His legs were skinny when they once were strong, he didn't know what day it was and could not remember the names of everyday objects. It was like he had Alzheimer's. He still recognized me and my mom, but other people depended. He really liked our dog. She was always very gentle around him and after he died we said where's daddy and she went to where his bed had been and looked around for him. That was so sad, we burst into tears. My uncle would come to see my dad and bring him a Big Mac every Monday. My aunt, his sister, never came to see him after he had started to look sick. Eventually he had to have a catheter put in, but he tried to pull it out. He was in pain all night. At the end he couldn't move. He just lay in bed. I don't think that he was in a coma, but he might have been. We had a birthday party for him on his 50th birthday. We made a giant cake and put 50 candles on it. We almost burnt the house down. He was aware enough to blow the candles out but didn't know the names of all the people that were there. He died only about a week or two weeks later. It was right after Halloween because I had gone to my friend's party and had to come home. My mom's parents were there and my mom and I was upstairs when he died. They called me down after he had died to say goodbye. I had been sitting in my room under two chairs that I had put a sheet over. People sent flowers and food. At the funeral me and my mom sat in the front row and each had a rose and put it on this stand that had his picture on it. My best friend wouldn't come, but every one else was there. My friends from school and my teacher came, my whole family and all of my dad's parents' friends whom I didn't know. There was food and I was playing around on the electric organ. The church was packed. We went home and all the flowers sat in our living room and throughout our house for weeks until they all slowly died. We spread my dad's ashes in the ocean on his friend's boat and all of his sailing friends were with us. I marked the location with the GPS of where we put his ashes into the ocean. We always used to go sailing on the weekends and it was the perfect way to remember him.

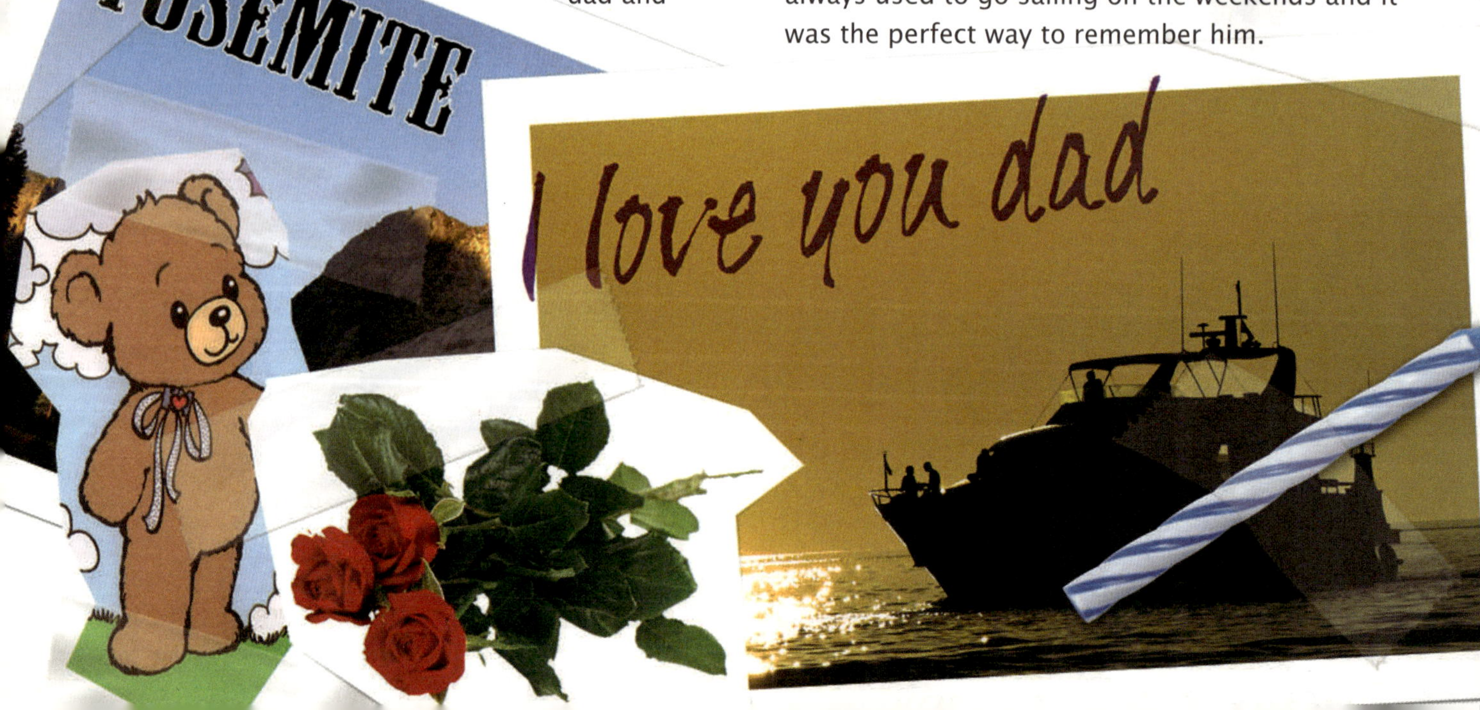

USE THIS PAGE

USE THIS PAGE

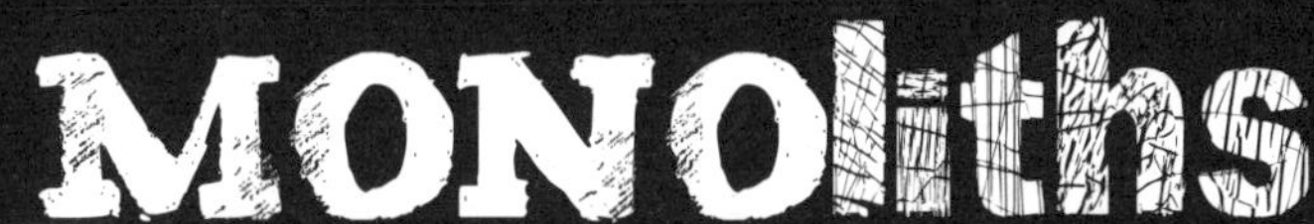

MONOliths

BY Wesley

CAN I DESTROY THE ROCK PILLARS?
WHERE ARE THESE SACRED MONOLITHS?
WHAT IS THAT WRITING ON THE WALL, MY KILLER?
WRITTEN IN BLOOD IS THIS:

You who shall see all that is naught
You who shall kill by your own creed
Here is the grave of which I sought
When you die you leave behind your deeds

THE SANDS OF SPACE REPENT
THE WATER OF TIME RIPPLES
HERE LIES INFINITY'S DECENT
IN LIFE, REALITY CRIPPLES

But in the silence of lost words
I will show you my capability
Fly above all of death's birds
I will show you your own hostility

BUT ON THE WALL OF THY PHARAOH
THE BLOOD-WORDS REMAIN
FALLEN IS YOUR ONLY HERO
TRAPPED IN THE FISSURE'S FAME

-2004

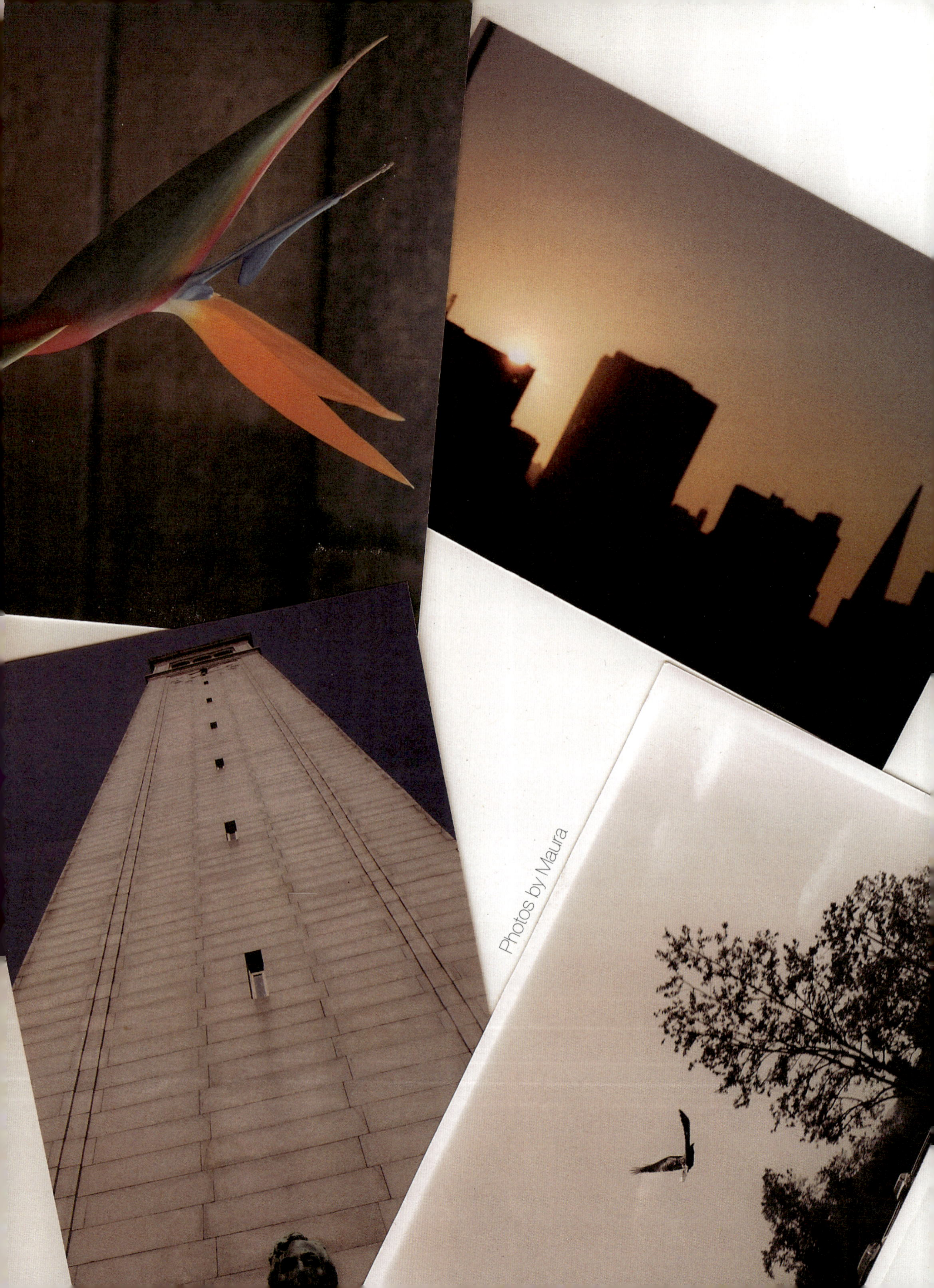
Photos by Maura

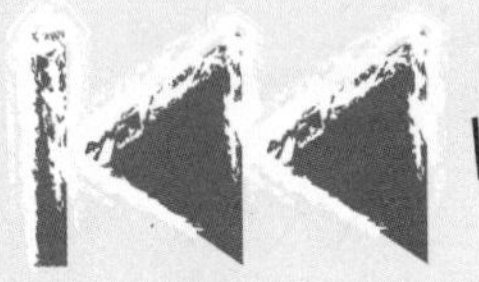

ESSAY BY MIRANDA

Wait, Rewind:

The year is 1995, and it's Thanksgiving Day. Everybody's filled up on Grandma's good food and the remains of a delicious meal are threatening to take over the picnic table. A man, slightly overweight, with black hair and a calm demeanor, is busy tickling his 5 year old daughter, as his 4 year old son is anxiously trying to join the fun too. Mom snaps a picture, capturing the memory forever.

Forward:

It's Christmas Day, 2006, and the same man is browsing through the fridge, this time with what his friends say is "a good weight for him" He has a little more salt and pepper in his hair, and a slight yellow tint to his skin, probably due to whatever it is that has been making him so sick lately. He feels a pang in his stomach, one that he later says, "would send any other person to the emergency room." But my dad isn't that person. He's never been the one to panic, choosing instead to rationalize and save worrying for another day, thinking it's just the stomach flu.

Ok, Play:

My dad has Pancreatic Cancer. At 54 years old, he is 6 feet tall, has thin frizzly hair, and is as skinny as me, his 17 year old daughter who weighs 115 pounds. There are a lot of things I could tell you, like how this cancer has a 99% mortality rate, or about the spots on his liver, or even how I spent an entire spring break in a hospital by his side. Either way, the fact still is: my dad is dying. And there isn't anything that hasn't been tried, to stop it. Unless you've been through it, you'll never understand the immense heartbreak of watching somebody you love face the end of their life before they should, of watching a hardworking man get too tired and dizzy to even stand up anymore. You'll never understand the agony of not knowing whether or not your father will get to see you graduate high school. But here is another fact: every single one of us is risking our lives constantly. Here I am, my heart ripped apart because at some point I'll lose my dad, when at any moment, I could lose my mother, one of my siblings, or a friend thanks to a car accident or some other tragic event, and not even know what hit me. We spend so much time fussing over the reasons our life isn't perfect, worrying about sadness we'll all end up feeling at various points, and never taking the time to look around us and see the beauty in what we have. I've spent hours and hours going over the "What If's" of all this. What if he had gone to the emergency room? What if Kaiser hadn't wasted so much time? And even ridiculous questions like, what if he had just eaten less soda and red meat? But the fact remains, my dad is still dying. Right now.

And right now, wasting time on questions that I can never answer, doesn't bring me any closer to understanding the how or the why. In fact, the how and the why isn't really what's important, and I'm not too sure it ever is. It is what it is, and as sad as it makes me, nothing is going to change the fact that my wonderful dad is sick. Overanalyzing every possible reason it all went wrong, doesn't change that it went wrong. It's still going wrong, but all I can do is love him and be thankful for the time I have with him, not agonize and try to change the past. I think this is something useful for every aspect of a person's life, not just a loved one being diagnosed with cancer. All I can ever do, in any part of my life, is roll with the punches and deal with things as they happen.

In a lot of ways, my dad's diagnosis and prognosis matured me very rapidly in a lot of ways. It was as if I was suddenly free of so many useless teenage worries and concerns, and everything I didn't need to feel just dissolved away. The ex-boyfriends, the self-consciousness, the stupid drama, the need to constantly fit in and be approved of . . . gone. I look around at my classmates now, hear their constant chatter about boys, girls, their hair, complaints about their parents, complaints about each other, and wonder how it can possibly be that they don't realize, it doesn't matter. None of it matters. The only thing that matters, and I think everybody eventually learns, is to love the people in your life, and the experiences you've had. Being happy with yourself and taking the time to enjoy things while you still have the chance. Eventually, all good things must come to pass. Whether it's my dad, my friends, the rest of my family, or anybody else that I love, eventually they won't be around anymore, and all that I'll have is the memories of everything we shared. Today is the day to be thankful. Today is the day to tell them you love them. Today is the day to make the most of the time you have. All I can ask for, all that anybody can ask for, is just another good day.

miranda :)))))))))))))))))

I have learned that even land locked lovers yearn

by wynne

I OFTEN WALK DOWN THE SIDEWALK OF MY UNIVERSITY CONFUSED ON HOW IT IS I GOT THERE. WHERE DID ALL THAT TIME GO? WHERE HAVE I TUCKED MY FRUSTRATION OF SO MANY YEARS AGO? AT EIGHTEEN YEARS OLD, I CAN SAY THIS PAST SEPTEMBER WAS THE FOURTH YEAR SINCE MY MOTHER'S DEATH FROM CANCER.

SHE DID NOT SEE ME NEARLY OVERDOSE ON COUGH SYRUP, SNEAK OUT A BROKEN WINDOW TO DO DRUGS WITH OTHER BROKEN PEOPLE, GRADUATE HIGH SCHOOL, ENTER COLLEGE, OR REMEMBER THAT I LOVED MY DAD.

IT IS ON THE SIDEWALK OF MY UNIVERSITY THAT I WONDER WHAT SHE WOULD THINK OF ME. ASIDE FROM LOVING WHATEVER I BECAME, I WONDER WHAT SHE WOULD THINK ABOUT THE SCHOOL MY DAD AND ME CHOSE. THE CLOTHING THAT I WEAR, THE ATTITUDE I HAVE, MY REPUTATION AT HOME, AND MY NEW ONE HERE AT SCHOOL.

ALWAYS A CURIOUS PHENOMENON, DEATH HAS HAUNTED NEARLY EVERYTHING THAT I DO. WHEN I GET TO KNOW SOMEONE AND I ADMIT TO THEM I AM MOTHERLESS, BUT I STILL HAVE A MOTHER. OR WHEN I TALK ABOUT MY PASSIONS, CANCER SUPPORT GROUPS. AND EVEN THOUGH IT HAS HAPPENED REPEATEDLY NOW, THE TEARS THAT CREEP DOWN MY CHEEKS WHEN WE LOSE ANOTHER MEMBER. I MIGHT BE USED TO DEATH BY NOW, BUT NO MATTER HOW MANY DIFFERENT PLACES I TRY TO PUT IT: MY STYLE, MY PERSONALITY, MY COLLEGE, MY STROLL ALONG THE SIDEWALK, IT IS NEVER A COMFORTABLE PART OF ME.

I HAVE TOLD OTHERS THAT THE PAIN NEVER STOPS, YOU JUST LEARN TO MAKE IT A PART OF YOUR LIFE. I NEGLECT TO ADMIT THAT ALONG WITH THAT NEW PAIN, IS NEW RESENTMENT, NEW SADNESS ALL IT'S OWN. RESENTFUL THAT YOU MUST BE FORCED TO LIVE WITH PAIN YOU DID NOT ASK FOR, DAILY SADNESS THAT OCCURS EVERY MORNING WHEN YOU WAKE UP AND ACKNOWLEDGE FOR THAT SPLIT SECOND THAT YOU ARE STILL IN THE SAME PAIN YOU WERE IN FOUR YEARS AGO.

DEATH DOES NOT ASK FOR YOUR PERMISSION, IT DOES NOT ASK FOR YOUR ACCEPTANCE. THOSE TWO THINGS YOU MUST CREATE FOR YOURSELF, AND IN DOING SO MUST DO ALONE.

Memories fade, but they do not disappear. Voices lose their clarity, but they still belong to you. The only thing that death cannot remove, not matter how cliché, is love.

AS A FOURTEEN YEAR OLD I TOLD MY MOM I WOULD KILL MYSELF IF SHE DIED. HORRIFIED, SHE TURNED TO ME AND ASKED ME TO REVOKE MY COMMENT. I WAS SERIOUS, ALTHOUGH AFTER SHE DIED FELT A DIFFERENT AND MORE RATIONAL SORT OF LOYALTY. MY MOTHER HAS NOT BECOME A SAINT AFTER HER DEATH, BUT THE LOVE AND LOYALTY I FELT FOR HER AS A CHILD, TEENAGER AND NOW ADULT, IS JUST AS STRONG AND BLAZING AS EVER.

Love doesn't care if death asks for permission or not, it is its own separate entity, to which you may always return to and claim.

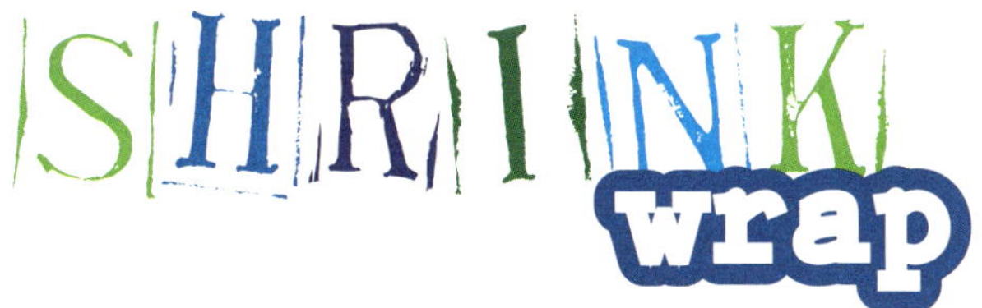

How do YOU cope?

With all this adversity in your life it can be difficult to cope, and what does coping mean anyways? Here is how the dictionary describes it:
a: to maintain a contest or combat usually on even terms or with success
b: to deal with and attempt to overcome problems and difficulties

How have you dealt with problems in the past and present? How do you combat the tough times? How do you find success in your life when all of "this" is happening? Here are some the responses our teens gave us as both healthy and unhealthy coping. The choice is yours to make.

The problem with the unhealthy choices is they inevitably add to your problem list. The healthy choices will make you feel better during your toughest times and can become the "thing" that gets you through, without adding more garbage to the pile.

- Lynnette

UNHEALTHY COPING

Denial that the problem exists.

Not talking about it.

Not telling your friends, etc.

Creating more chaos in your life. (for example: ditching class, skipping soccer practice, etc.)

Self Mutilation

Compulsive Eating

Drug & Alcohol Use and Abuse

Sleeping Excessively

Running Away

Spacing Out

Anorexia/Bulimia

Shoplifting

HEALTHY COPING

Listening to Music

Hanging out with friends that are a good influence on you and are supportive of what you are going through

Being home, being helpful, staying involved

Spending time with your parent who has cancer. Especially if your parent's diagnosis is grave, this is precious time together. Avoid your impulse to bail out......stay close.

Exercise/Sports

Writing in a Journal

Getting a Job

Staying on top of school work/ Avoiding the stress of being behind and playing catch up

Talking to my parents/friends.....or even a therapist about how this is affecting me

Going to a Kids Konnected Support Group

GLOSSARY

BENIGN Harmless; not cancerous

BIOPSY The removal of cells or tissues to help identify disease. There are 3 types of biopsies:

1. Incisional or core: Just a sample of tissue is removed.
2. Needle or fine needle-aspiration: A sample of tissue or fluid is removed with a needle.
3. Excisional: A whole tumor or lesion is removed.
4. Bone scan: A radiologic scan of the skeleton, used to detect bone metastasis.

CANCER A general term for more than one hundred diseases that are characterized by uncontrolled, abnormal growth of cells.

CANCER STAGING When a cancer diagnosis is made, a stage is assigned to aid in selecting the appropriate course of treatment and determining the prognosis. There are four primary stages (I, II, III and IV) and subcategories for different situations.

There are several factors that are taken into account, typically using the TNM model:

T stands for the tumor size.
N stands for whether or not the cancer has spread to nearby lymph nodes.
M stands for whether or not the cancer has metastasized.

The higher the stage number, the more advanced the cancer is. For example, a Stage IV cancer would have metastasized to more than one organ and to nearby lymph nodes.

COMPAZINE (generic name: prochlorperazine): A drug that helps control nausea and vomiting after surgery or chemotherapy.

CT SCAN Computed tomography (CT) scans, also called CAT scans, are a radiographic technique that uses a computer to assimilate multiple x-ray images into a two-dimensional cross-sectional image.

CYST A nodule that is filled with fluid and is typically benign.

ETIOLOGY The cause and origins of diseases.

MARGINS The area of tissue that surrounds a tumor when it is removed by surgery. The term "clean margins" is used to describe tissue that does not contain cancer cells and indicates that all the cancer has been removed. The term "dirty margins" is a term used when the tissue removed contains cancer cells, and is indicative of cancer remaining in the tissue after surgery.

METASTASES (METASTATIC) The spread of cancer from the primary location of the cancer (such as the

GLOSSARY

breast) to other locations in the body (such as the bones, lungs, liver or brain).

NADIR During cancer treatment, when measuring blood counts, this is the point at which the blood counts are at their lowest point. The patient is considered immune repressed.

NEO-ADJUVANT Treatment, usually chemotherapy, radiation or hormones that are given first, before surgery with the goal of helping make the next step of treatment go more smoothly. It is used often in breast cancer to shrink a large tumor so that later on it's easier to remove surgically.

OCCLUDED Blocked or closed.

ONCOLOGIST A physician who specializes in the diagnosis and treatment of patients with cancer. A "medical oncologist" specializes in the treatment of cancer through the use of chemotherapy drugs. A "radiation oncologist" specializes in the treatment of cancer through the use of radiotherapy measures.

PALLIATIVE Measures taken to provide relief to the patient, but not meant to cure the condition.

PATHOLOGY REPORT A written report that summarizes the studies performed on tissue removed from the body, either through surgery or a biopsy. The information in the report is used to determine the best treatment options.

PORT-A-CATH A brand name for the type of small catheter device that is placed on the chest, under the skin and into a blood vessel making it easier to give chemotherapy and to take blood tests. Also called a "central line."

PROPHYLACTIC A preventive measure, such as surgery or medication, to decrease the likelihood of a cancer recurrence or the development of cancer in a particular location.

RADIATION PORTAL The area where external radiation enters the body.

RECONSTRUCTION The rebuilding or repairing of an area of the body that has been damaged or removed.

RECURRENCE When cancer returns after treatment. Cancer may return to the same original cancer site (local recurrence) or in a different part of the body (metastatic recurrence).

REMISSION A decrease in or disappearance of the signs and symptoms of cancer. Partial remission is the disappearance of some but not all signs and symptoms of cancer. Complete remission is the disappearance of all signs and symptoms, although cancer cells may still be present in the body.

GLOSSARY

TREATMENTS

Surgery – The removal of a tumor by cutting it out of the body.

Radiation – The use of high-energy radiation or high-energy particles to control or cure cancer. It may reduce the size of a cancer before surgery or be used to destroy any remaining cancer cells after surgery. It can also be helpful in treating recurrent cancers or relieving symptoms. Radiation may come from a machine (external beam radiation therapy), or it may come from radioactive material placed in the body in the area near cancer cells (internal radiation therapy). Radiation is also called radiotherapy.

Chemotherapy – Medication used to kill cells that are rapidly reproducing. These medications kill both cancerous (unhealthy) and noncancerous (healthy) cells. There is also a type of chemotherapy that is called "targeted therapy," these drugs are less toxic to healthy cells, targeting only the cancer cells. The drugs can be given as a pill, an injection or shot or through an IV (intravenously).

Stem cell transplantation – A procedure that uses stem cells which are found in one's bone marrow or blood to restore stem cells that have been destroyed by chemotherapy or radiation therapy.

Hormone Therapy – A treatment that takes advantage of the tendency of some cancers to stabilize or shrink if certain hormones are added, blocked or removed.

Biological Therapy – A treatment that affects tumors indirectly by stimulating the immune system to fight cancer. Examples of drugs used are: interferon, IL-2 and LAK cells.

TUMOR BOARD A panel of medical experts who discuss a patient's diagnosis and make cancer treatment recommendations.

ULTRASOUND A type of imaging technique that uses high-frequency sound waves to take pictures of internal organs.

ZOFRAN (generic name, ondansetron HCl): A drug that helps relieve nausea and vomiting associated with chemotherapy or surgery.

The glossary definitions were taken from information on the following websites:

- **www.breastcancer.org**
- **www.cancerweb.ncl.ac.uk**
- **www.komen.org**
- **www.cancer.org**
- **www.imaginis.com**
- **www.cancergroup.com**
- **www.nci.gov**

CONTENTMENT IS NOT
THE FULFILLMENT OF WHAT
YOU WANT, BUT THE
REALIZATION OF HOW MUCH
YOU ALREADY HAVE.

ANONYMOUS

Alabama

Bosom Buddies: Cullman Regional Medical Center, Cullman, AL• (256) 737-2630
• General Cancer Support Groups

Wilma Ruffin: Normal, AL • (256) 372-4960
• General Cancer Support Groups

Alaska

Currently no groups, please check cancerconnected.com for updated listings.

Arizona

Children to Children: (520) 322-9155
• Support for kids with a parent or relative with cancer

Banner Good Samaritan Medical Center:
1111 E. McDowell Road,
Phoenix, AZ 85006 • (602) 239-2000
• Support groups for Kids – "Kids Connect" (602) 239-5909

Banner Thunderbird Medical Center:
5555 W. Thunderbird Road, Glendale, AZ 85306 (602) 865-5555
• Kids Can Cope: This free group focuses on the needs of children, ages 6-16, who are coping with a relative or friend's cancer diagnosis. The group meets 6:30 to 8 p.m. on the first and third Tuesday of each month in the Radiation Oncology conference room, located in Outpatient Services. For more information and specific directions, please call Patti Jensen at (602) 865-5450.

Bosom Buddies: Phoenix, AZ
(480) 661-6228 or (480) 998-8592
• Support for kids with a parent or relative with cancer

The Family Circle Group:
Phoenix, AZ • (602) 712-1006
• Support groups for kids with a parent or relative with cancer

Arkansas

HOPE, Inc.: 2949 Point Circle, Suite 1, Fayetteville, AR 72704
• CLIMB® Program – The CLIMB® Program at is a support group for children who have parents with cancer. The program is for children ages 7-14 and meets once a week for six weeks. For more information about upcoming CLIMB® programs, please call (479) 571-4673.

Northwest Cancer Support Home:
Fayetteville, AR • (479) 521-8024
• General Cancer Support Groups

CARTI Cancer Awareness:
Little Rock, AR • (800) 482-8561
• One-on-one counseling for kids who have a parent with cancer. Email: owyatt@carti.com or visit www.carti.com

California

Kids Konnected: Laguna Hills, CA
(949) 582-5443 or (800) 899-1288
www.kidskonnected.org
• Support Services for Kids who have a Parent with Cancer. Support Groups, Summer Camps, Teddy Bear Outreach, Youth Leadership Program.

Brea, CA – Kids Konnected Support Group: Meets the fourth Tuesday of each month from 6:30-8:00 p.m. at the Brea Community Center, Meeting Room H, 695 Madison Ave., Brea, CA 92821.
Call for info: (949) 582-5443

Mission Viejo, CA – Kids Konnected Support Group: Meets the second Monday of each month from 6:30-8:00 p.m. at the Mission Hospital Conference Center, 26726 Crown Valley Pkwy. Call: (949) 582-5443.

Newport Beach, CA – Kids Konnected Support Group: Meets the 1st and 3rd Monday of each month. Separate groups for ages 4 to 6, 7 to 12, Teens and Parents. Meetings are held from 7:00-8:00 p.m. Pizza from 6:30-7:00 p.m. at the Hoag Cancer Center in Newport Beach.
Call for info: (949) 582-5443.

Orange, CA – Kids Konnected Support Group: Meets the 2nd and 4th Tuesday of each month from 7:00-8:00 p.m. Cordelia Knott Center for Wellness, 230 South Main Street, Suite 210. Call: (949) 582-5443.

San Diego, CA - Kids Konnected Support Group: Meets the second Thursday of each month from 7:00-8:00 p.m. at The Scripps Mende Well Being Center - 4305 La Jolla Village Dr, Suite L-5 (above Peking Restaurant) University Towne Center.

Santa Clara, CA - Kids Konnected Support Group: Group meets the 1st and 3rd Tuesday of each month from 6:30-8:00 p.m. at Parents Helping Parents, 3041 Olcott St., Santa Clara, 95054. Please RSVP by calling (408) 496-6336.

Temecula/Murrieta, CA - Kids Konnected Support Group: NEW LOCATION! Meetings held at Michelle's Place 41785 Elm St., Suite 305, Murrieta (Second building in from Elm St). Meets the 2nd Tuesday of each month from 6:30-7:30 p.m. No RSVP necessary. Just show up! If you have any questions call (949) 582-5443 for more info.

Art & Creativity For Healing Inc.
Laguna Niguel, CA • (949) 367-1902
• Art Workshops for kids and adults www.art4healing.org

Long Beach Memorial Breast Center:
Long Beach, CA • (562) 933-7880
or (562) 933-0900
• Support groups for kids with a parent or relative with cancer

City of Hope – Duarte, CA
(626) 256-8626
www.cityofhope.org
• Kids Konnected Support Group

Center for Psychology of Cancer
Newport Beach, CA • (949) 474-4337
• One-on-one counseling for kids who have a parent with cancer

Circle of Care: Oakland, CA
(510) 531-7551
• Support groups for kids with a parent or relative with cancer

Kara: Palo Alto, CA • (650) 321-5272
• Support groups for kids with a parent with cancer

The Wellness Community-Pasadena:
Pasadena, CA • (626) 796-1083
• Cancer Support Groups

Center for Attitudinal Healing:
Sausalito, CA • (415) 331-6161
• Support groups for kids with a parent with cancer

We Spark:
Sherman Oaks, CA • (818) 906-3022
• Support groups for kids with a parent with cancer

The Wellness Community:
Walnut Creek, CA • (925) 933-0107
• Support groups for kids with a parent with cancer

Kids Can Cope: (323) 564-7911
• Support groups for kids with a parent with cancer.

Cancer Resources

Colorado

The Tree House: Grand Junction, CO
territreehouse@aol.com • (970) 241-8001
• Support groups for kids

University of Colorado Cancer Center:Anschutz Cancer Pavilion
1665 N. Ursula St. Aurora, CO 80045
• Children's Lives Include Moments of Bravery (C.L.I.M.B.), is a support group for children to help them cope with a parent or caregivers cancer. Call Lori McKeon at (720) 848-0249.

The Children's Treehouse Foundation:
Denver, CO • (303) 322-1202
www.childrenstreehousefdn.org
• Children's Lives Include Moments of Bravery (C.L.I.M.B.) is a six-week-long program for children with a parent with cancer.

Wellness Center at McKee Medical Center:
Loveland, CO
• Hearts of Hope – a regional support program for children ages 7-16 who have loved ones with cancer. Meetings are held one Saturday per month from 9:00-11:00 a.m.
Call (970) 635-4129 for meeting dates.

Connecticut

Middlesex Hospital Cancer Center
536 Saybrook Road, Middletown, CT 06457
(860) 358-6763 or (860) 344-6000
• Children's Lives Include Moments of Bravery (C.L.I.M.B.) For children with parents or grandparents with cancer.
Email: Wendy_Peterson@midhosp.org

Ann's Place - The Home of I Can
Danbury, CT • (203) 790-6568
• Cancer Support Groups
• Family Action Network
• Short-term family counseling following new diagnosis.

The Center for Hope:
Darien, CT • (203) 655-4693
• Cancer Support Groups

Cancer Care, Inc.
Norwalk, CT • (800) 813-HOPE (4673)
• Cancer Support Groups

Delaware

Please see listings for New Jersey. Check cancerconnected.com for updates.

Florida

Moffitt Cancer Center (MCC)
12902 Magnolia Drive, Tampa, FL 33612
(813) 745-4673
• Families First helps parents and their children as they adjust to the changes that occur within the family when a parent has cancer. Information, preparation and support enable families to cope successfully in the face of a serious illness.

Please contact the Psychosocial & Palliative Care Program Office at (813) 745-8407 for assistance with community resources.

Rainbows: Fort Myers, FL • (239) 334-7797
• Bereavement groups for kids
email: GELARDIJ@STFRACIS2055.com

Georgia

Georgia Cancer Specialists
• Children's Lives Include Moments of Bravery (C.L.I.M.B.) is a six-week-long program for children with a parent with cancer.
To register, contact Lisa Andreucci, LCSW (770) 496-9489 ext. 320, or Jennifer McNeilly, LMSW (770) 496-9489 ext. 210.

The Cancer Center at DeKalb Medical:
Atlanta, GA • (404) 501-EASY (3279)
• Tree House Gang - Support Groups for Kids who have a Parent with Cancer

Kids Cope: Atlanta, GA • www.kidscope.org
• Cancer Support Resources

Hawaii

American Cancer Society – East Hawaii Unit Hilo, HI • (808) 935-9763
www.cancer.org
• Support groups for kids

American Cancer Society – West Hawaii Unit Kailua-Kona, HI • (808) 334-0442
• Support resources for kids
email: tchlothie@cancer.org

American Cancer Society – Kauai Unit
Lihue, HI • (808) 245-2942
Support resources for kids

American Cancer Society – Maui Unit
Wailukku, HI • (808) 244-5553
• Support groups for kids
email: mauiunit@cancer.org

Idaho

St. Luke's Wellness Watch:
Boise, ID • (800) 845-4624 or (208) 381-3161
• Support groups for kids

Illinois

Kids Konnected: www.kidskonnected.org
Peoria, IL: Kids Konnected Support Group: Kids ages 5-18 meet the 1st and 3rd Monday of every month at the Holt Education Center. Call for info: (888) 566-3653

Rainbows:
Rolling Meadows, IL • (847) 925-1770
• Bereavement groups for kids
email: SUZY@RAINBOWS.ORG

Indiana

Kids Konnected: www.kidskonnected.org
Greater Lafayette, IN, Kids Konnected Support Group: Group meets on the 2nd Monday of each month, 6:00-7:30 p.m. at First Christian Church, 329 North 6th Street, Lafayette. Call Jane Anderson for info: (765) 497-3516. You can visit their website at www.kidskonnectedin.org

Wellness Community
Indianapolis, IN • (317) 257-1505
• Cancer Support Groups

Health Ministry Partnership
Mishawaka, IN • (574) 254-0454 ext. 202
• Bereavement groups for kids
email: CLEMANSB@SBIENT.COM

Iowa

Siouxland Regional Cancer Center
Sioux City, IA • (712) 252-9338
• Support resources for kids

Kansas

Please see listings for Oklahoma. Check cancerconnected.com for updates.

Kentucky

Please see listings for Tennessee. Check cancerconnected.com for updates.

Cancer Resources

Louisiana

Kathy Stelly: Lafayette, LA
(337) 261-5551
• Cancer Support Groups
email: Kathy@dol-louisiana.org

Ochsner Cancer Center
New Orleans, LA • (504) 842-5200
• Cancer Support Groups

Maine

Breast Cancer Support Group
Caribou, ME • (207) 498-3111
• Support groups for kids

Maryland

Upper Chesapeake Medical Center
500 Upper Chesapeake Drive,
Bel Air, MD 21014 • (443) 643-1000
• Children's Lives Include Moments of Bravery (C.L.I.M.B.), is a support group for children to help them cope with a parent or caregivers cancer.

Wellness Community:
Baltimore, MD • (410) 832-2719
• Cancer Support Groups

Massachusetts

The Wellness Community
Newton, MA • (617) 332-1919
www.wellnesscommunity.org
• For information about other Wellness Communities in the U.S. and abroad, go to www.thewellnesscommunity.org.

• Kids Count Too – Cancer Support Groups

Dana-Farber/Brigham and Women's Cancer Center: Boston, MA
Department of Care Coordination at (617) 632-3301
or e-mail: familyconnections@dfci.harvard.edu
• Family Connection Program provides support resources for kids

Lowell General Hospital
295 Varnum Ave., Lowell, MA 01854
• A support group for teens ages 14 to 17 who have been affected by cancer in their family. Meets the second Tuesday of each month from 3:30-4:30 p.m. Please call Cammie Caron at 978-937-6129 to register.

Rainbows Webster, MA • (508) 943-0953
• Bereavement groups for kids
email: MSLRAINBOWS@AOL.COM

Michigan

Connie Gladhill:
Allen Park, MI • (313) 383-2353
• Cancer Support Groups
email: rainbows@surfmk.com

Alexander J. Walt Breast Center
Detroit, MI • (800) KARMANOS
• Cancer Support Groups

Gilda's Club Metro Detroit:
Royal Oak, MI • (248) 577-0800 ext. 31
• Cancer Support Groups

Minnesota

American Cancer Society
2520 Pilot Knob Rd, Ste 150
Mendota Heights, MN 55120 • (651) 255-8100
• Cancer resources and referrals.

Mississippi

Please see listings for Louisiana. Check cancerconnected.com for updates.

Missouri

Missouri Baptist Medical Center
3015 North Ballas Road, St. Louis, Missouri 63131 • (314) 996-5000
• Bear Essentials: A support group for children 4-12 years old who have a parent with cancer. For more information, please call (314) 996-5517.

Montana

Northern Rockies Cancer Center
Billings, MT • (406) 248-2212
• Cancer Support Groups

St. Peter's Hospital
Helena, MT • (406) 444-2381
• Cancer Support Groups

Nebraska

Family Life Circle
Omaha, NE • (402) 551-3050
• Bereavement groups for kids
email: jgould@omahaflo.creighton.edu

Nevada

Kids Konnected: www.kidskonnected.org

Las Vegas, Nevada – Kids Konnected Support Group: Meets the 1st and 3rd Tuesday of each month from 7:00-8:00 p.m. at the Nevada Childhood Cancer Foundation Center, 6070 S. Eastern Ave. For more info and to RSVP contact Rosalie Montoya MSW, LCSW at 702-371-0046. This location is generously sponsored to us by the Nevada Community Foundation.

Sparks, Nevada - Kids Konnected Support Group: Meets the 2nd Monday of each month at the Spanish Springs Library, 7100A pyramid Lake Highway (located in Lazy 5 Regional Park, Sparks, Nevada 89436, phone (775) 424-1800. We will be meeting from 6:30-8:00 p.m. in the Washoe room. The therapist name is Laurie Drucker, Psy.D. (775) 323-2255.

New Hampshire

Please see listings for Massachusetts. Check cancerconnected.com for updates.

New Jersey

The Wellness Community
3 Crossroads Dr., Bedminster, NJ 07921
(908) 658-5400
email: centralnj@thewellnesscommunity.org
• Teens Connect - Monthly program for teens who have a parent diagnosed with cancer. Meets on Thursday evenings.

New Mexico

People living though Cancer
Albuquerque, NM • (505) 242-3263
• Cancer Support Groups

Y-ME of Southern New Mexico
Las Cruces, NM • (504) 524-4373
• Cancer Support Groups

New York

Kids Konnected: www.kidskonnected.org

New York, NY - Kids Konnected Support Group: SHARE at the Jewish Community Center in Manhatten. Call (866) 891-2392 for info. Kids ages 7-13 meet two Saturdays a month from 11:30 a.m.-1:00 p.m.

Cancer Resources

New York

Cancer Care, Inc.
New York, NY • (800) 813-HOPE (4673)
• Cancer Support Groups

Memorial Sloan Kettering Cancer Center
New York, NY
• Individual and family counseling, offered through the Department of Psychiatry, may also be helpful. To contact the Department of Psychiatry, call 646-888-0100.

North Carolina

Rex Hospital — Main Campus
4420 Lake Boone Trail
Raleigh, NC, 27607 • (919) 784-3100
• Kidscan!, a monthly support group program sponsored by the Holt Foundation, is specifically designed for children ages 6-12 to help them understand their parent or loved ones' cancer. Please call (919) 784-6455 for more information.

St. Andrew The Apostle Church
Apex, NC • (919) 362-0685 ext. 25
• Cancer Support Groups
email: quintal@wave-net.net

North Dakota

Trinity Medical Center
West Minot, ND • (701) 857-5265
• Cancer Support Groups

Ohio

Ohio State University Comprehensive Cancer Center – James Cancer Hospital and Solove Research Institute (OSUCCC - James)
300 W. 10th Ave.; Columbus, Ohio 43210
1-800-293-5066
• Kaleidoscope - A teen group led by a licensed art therapist. Creative art interventions such as photography, journaling, painting and several other types of expressive arts modalities are used to help teens express complicated emotions and fear. Meets Thursday evenings from 6:30-8:00 p.m. for 6 weeks. For more information or to register, send us an email with your name, phone number and address or call us at (614) 293-4138.
• Anger in Motion (A.I.M.): Led by a licensed art therapist who indulges the express their anger through sports, these teens learn ways to cope with their anger and deal with their fears and emotions due to the illness or death in the family. Meets Thursday evenings from 6:30-8:00 p.m. for 6 weeks. For more information or to register, send us an email with your name, phone number and address or call us at (614) 293-4138.

Oklahoma

Kids Konnected: www.kidskonnected.org.
Oklahoma City, OK - Kids Konnected Support Group: Kids ages 7-17 meet the 1st Thursday of every month at 6:30 p.m. in St.Anthony's Hospital. Call (405) 623-4997 for information.

Oregon

Kids Konnected: www.kidskonnected.org
Medford, OR - Kids Konnected Support Group: Kids ages 4-17 meet the fourth Tuesday of every month from 6:30-8:00 p.m. at the First Methodist Church. Call Shelley Bailey for info call (541) 601-5935.

Providence Portland Medical Center
4805 NE Glisan Street, Portland, OR 97213
• Family Support Group: Meets the second Thursday of each month. Dinner is served from 6-6:30 p.m., followed by group from 6:30-8:00 p.m. Providence Professional Plaza, 5050 NE Hoyt, Level B. Children and teens that have a family member diagnosed with cancer benefit from a safe environment in which they can express their feelings. Groups are divided by age, with a parent group meeting at the same time. Please call Krista Nelson, MSW, at (503) 215-3204. Registration is required for this group.

Pennsylvania

Kids Konnected: www.kidskonnected.org
Reading, PA – Kids Konnected Support Group: Meets the fourth Monday of each month. Contact Christine Wasser at (610) 208-8830 for time and location.

York Cancer Center
York, PA • (877) 441-7957
• Kids Under Construction: This is a special support group for children who have parents with cancer. Call Barbara Titansih for information at (717) 993-6007.

Rhode Island

Please see listings for Massachusetts. Check cancerconnected.com for updates.

South Carolina

Please see listings for North Carolina. Check cancerconnected.com for updates.

South Dakota

Vera Sacred Heart Hospital
501 Summit Yankton, SD 57078
• CLIMB® Program – The CLIMB® Program at is a support group for children who have parents with cancer. The program is for children ages 7-14 and meets once a week for six weeks. Please call the Cancer Center at (605) 668-8850.

Tennessee

Kids Konnected: www.kidskonnected.org
Chattanooga, TN – Kids Konnected Support Group: Kids ages 7-13 meet the 3rd Thursday of each month at Erlanger Health Center in Administration building. Call Sam Harris at (423) 778-5119.

Gilda's Club Nashville
Nashville, TN • (615) 329-1124
• Cancer Support Groups for Patients and Family.

Texas

MD Anderson Cancer Center
1515 Holcombe Blvd, Houston, TX 77030
1-800-392-1611
• CLIMB (Children's Lives Include Moments of Bravery) CLIMB is a 6-week support group for children whose parents have cancer. Call Marisa at (713) 792-6826 for meeting times/dates and to determine eligibility.

Presbyterian Hospital of Dallas
8200 Walnut Hill Lane Dallas, TX 75231
214-345-6789
• CLIMB® Program – The CLIMB® Program at is a support group for children who have parents with cancer. The program is for children ages 7-14 and meets once a week for six weeks. Call (214) 345-6959.

Utah

Cancer Wellness House
Salt Lake City, UT • (801) 263-2294
• Cancer Support Groups

Vermont

Rutland Regional Medical Center:
160 Allen Street, Rutland, VT 05701
(802) 775-7111 RRMC Community Cancer Center.
• CLIMB® Program – The CLIMB® Program at is a support group for children who have parents with cancer. The program is for children ages 7 to 14 and meets once a week for six weeks. For more information please call Erica at (802) 747-1693.

Virginia

Inova Health System Life With Cancer Family Center
Fairfax, VA • (703) 208-5611
• Support Group for Teens.

Guild House, Lee's Friends: Helping People Live with Cancer
Norfolk, VA • (757) 625-3115
• General Support Groups

Washington

Kids Konnected: www.kidskonnected.org

Seattle, WA - Kids Konnected Support Group: Meetings held 2nd and 4th Tues of each month: 6:00pm-8:00pm at the World Harvester Family Church, 20830 52nd. Ave. West, Lynnwood, WA 98036 contact Sheila Wilson 206-227-0997

Bellevue, WA - Kids Konnected Support Group: Meets the first and third Tuesday of each month at Lincoln Center, 515 116th Ave. NE. Call Shelia Wilson for more details (206) 227-0997.

Bellingham, WA - Kids Konnected Support Group: Meets the third Monday of each month from 7:00-8:00 p.m. at St. Joseph's Cancer Center, 3217 Squalicum Pkwy. For more info contact Elizabeth Snyder, MS, LMHC (306) 739-5575.

Washington DC

Please see listings for Maryland or Virginia. Check cancerconnected.com for updates.

West Virginia

Please see listings for Virginia. Check cancerconnected.com for updates.

Wisconsin

Stillwaters Center, Inc.
434 Madison Street, Waukesha, WI 53188
Phone (262) 548-9148
• Children's Support Groups. For information call (262) 548-9148 or email us at inbox@stillwaterscenter.org

Wyoming

Please see listings for Colorado. Check cancerconnected.com for updates.

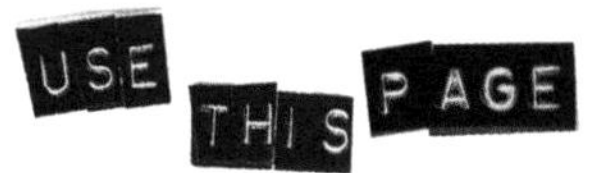
USE THIS PAGE

Short bio's for Contributing TEEN WRITERS

My name is Grady.
My mother died of breast cancer in November of 1997 when I was nine years old. Shortly after her death I started to attend a Kids Konnected support group. I have a younger sister and brother named Maura and Conor, and my Dad's name is Martin. I am currently attending college and pursuing a degree in Youth, Adult and Family Services, with hopes of getting a degree in Social work. I play the guitar and spend my time doing that instead of my school work.

My name is Maura.
I am a senior in High School. I began attending Kids Konnected support groups after my mom died from breast cancer. I later became a Youth Leader as I enjoyed helping the younger kids in the program.

My name is Conor.
I'm a sophomore in High School. My mother died from breast cancer when I was only 5 years old. I have an older brother and sister. I have a passion for gymnastics and hope to be in the Olympics some day.

My name is Cole.
I am a student at a university in the North East where I am studying Mechanical Engineering. I became involved with Kids Konnected as a sophomore in High School. I felt drawn to the organization, because when I was in fifth grade my Mom was diagnosed with Thyroid cancer and had her thyroid removed shortly afterward. Thankfully, she is doing well today.

My name is Lydia.
I was born and raised in Texas, with my mother working in television and my father doing cinematography, but we moved to Indiana, when I was 18. I also have a younger sister and brother. My mother was diagnosed with breast cancer the first time when I was 17 and got a lumpectomy, and the second time when I was 20 and had to get a mastectomy. I am passionate about music, writing, laughing and shamelessly correcting peoples' grammar and linguistics. Also, very passionate about my dog, Moose.

My name is Wynne.
I'm a nineteen year old college freshman in the Midwest. I grew up in Indiana and both my parents worked at a local university, and I attended kindergarten, grade, middle and high school in the local area.
My mom was diagnosed in 1994 with an unknown type of cancer, I was five at the time. Growing up, my mom couldn't always do what other moms did, she didn't always have the energy or the time, as she continued to work full time as a professor and be a single mom for at least half of her illness. She never let those obstacles stop her, however, and made it an important part of her life to travel, work to your fullest, and indulge in luxuries. My mom lost her nine year battle with cancer in September 2003, surrounded by family and friends after having just returned less than a week before from delivering a key note speech at a Child Care conference in Scotland. She is an important part of my life still five years later. She would be very proud of me and my peers contribution to this fantastic book!

My name is Hayden.
My father died from melanoma when I was 14 years old. I started attending Kids Konnected support groups when my Dad was first diagnosed and later became a Youth Leader. I am currently in my 4th year of college in northern California.

My name is Brendan.
My mother died when I was 16 from lung cancer. She was not a smoker. I now live with my Dad and his fiancé and my sister. I am a senior in high school and enjoy cheerleading.

My name is Jennifer.
I'm a senior in high school and play volleyball. I also volunteer for Kids Konnected and many other non-profit organizations in my free time. My father was diagnosed with cancer when I was 10 and died when I was 11. I was very close to my father and will always miss him dearly. I enjoy staying busy with school and training my dog, shopping, and watching movies.

My name is Devon.
I live in the North West where I attend High School. My mother is a breast cancer survivor.

My name is Erika.
My father died from lung cancer when I was 14 years old. I started going to Kids Konnected support groups with my two younger sisters when he was first diagnosed. I later became a Youth Leader. During high school I enjoyed playing water polo. I am currently in my second year of college in northern California.

My name is Allison.
My father died from lung cancer. I started going to Kids Konnected support groups with my sisters when he was first diagnosed. Currently I'm in high school and enjoy playing the piano.

My name is Jessica.
I'm a freshman in college in the Northeast majoring in architectural engineering. When I was in eighth grade, my father was diagnosed with brain cancer. After a difficult struggle, he passed away after my freshmen year of high school. Currently I live with my mother and her younger brother. I love the beach in the summer and snowboarding in the winter. I also enjoy spending time with my friends and family and miss my father more with each passing day.

My name is Nick.
I live in the Northwest where I enjoy being in the outdoors, camping and dirt bike riding. I came to Kids Konnected when I was 12 years old after my mom was diagnosed with breast cancer.

My name is Zack.
I live in Southern California and am a Sophomore in High School.

My name is Justin.
When I was 16 my mom was diagnosed with stage 3, Follicular Lymphoma. The doctor said she was completely covered, from head to toe, with cancer. They really didn't think she would live long, and I remember thinking how I would lose her forever. After a seemingly never-ending battle, and truck loads of prayers, my mom is in remission now. There is no sign of it now, however it's not curable... so I trust in God. I'm now working at a marketing company in the Northwest as a customer service associate who fixes problems, and helps people. I'm also a diver. I love to scuba dive, snorkel, and want to start taking ocean and sealife pictures and be a photographer as well. In addition to being a diver, I'm also a student pilot, and love to fly...so I get the best of both worlds. A major hobby of mine is music. I love to play anything I can get my hands on. So far I've picked up the piano, guitar, bass, drums, and trumpet. I'm working on the sax now... I can't read notes, but I can play almost anything I hear, and I love it. I can express my emotion in music, in a way I can't even describe.

My name is Kelly. I was born in southern California and have continued to live here since then. I live with my younger sister and my dad. My mother died of a brain tumor in 2001 while I was in 4th grade. Although times have been hard, I have been able to conquer many of the obstacles that come with being a "motherless daughter" with the support of my friends, family, and Kids Konnected. I love listening to all kinds of music, watching movies, writing in my journal daily, and reading novels.

My name is Wesley.
My father was diagnosed with lymphoma when I was 9 years old. He is currently in remission. I enjoy playing a variety of instruments and making music and playing video games.

My name is Christina and I am a sophomore at high school. I have 2 sisters, an older one and a younger one. My mom is an ovarian cancer survivor. I am a good student and love to play soccer.

My name is Sarah and I have been a part of Kids Konnected since January of 1994 when my father was fighting the battle of pancreatic cancer and then passed away that March. Having Kids Konnected in my life made me realize that every moment was special and that I was not alone. Again in 2004 I was faced with cancer when my mom was diagnosed with breast cancer. With the skill that Kids Konnected gave me I knew that I could survive anything that was thrown my way. I currently live in southern California with my husband and continue to help Kids Konnected in every way possible.

My name is Miranda
I'm 17 years old. I was born and live in southern California with my mom and dad, my brothers Shane and Christian, and our silly poodle Truman. My dad was diagnosed with Pancreatic Cancer in April of 2007, the end of my junior year in high school. Things have been up and down since then, but mostly we are just trying to get by. I graduate this year and after that I will be working and attending the local community college.

Shrink Wrap Doc

Lynnette Wilhardt is a licensed clinical oncology social worker, who specializes in working with families who have a parent with cancer. She has a private practice in Orange County, California. She is also the Clinical Director for Kids Konnected, a non-profit organization that provides support, education, friendship and understanding to kids who have a parent with cancer.

Lynnette shares her passion for travel and adventure with her twin daughters Caitlin and Ashley, who are an endless source of love and joy. She is also blessed with her mother, Dolly and sisters Linda, Loretta and Leanne whose love and support have gotten there through some tough times and her best friend Steve who has shown her that unconditional love really does exist.

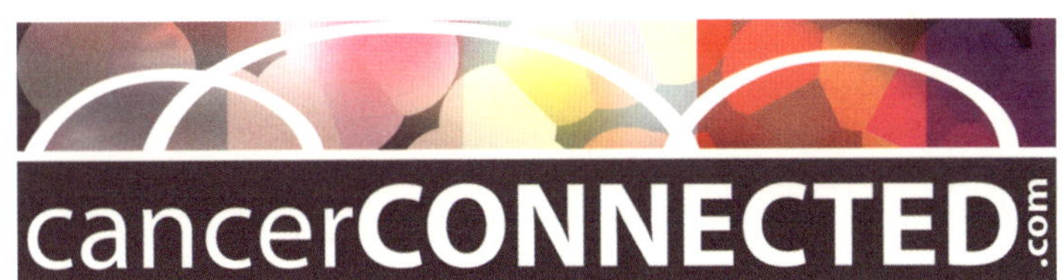

connect with other teens

•

share your creative work

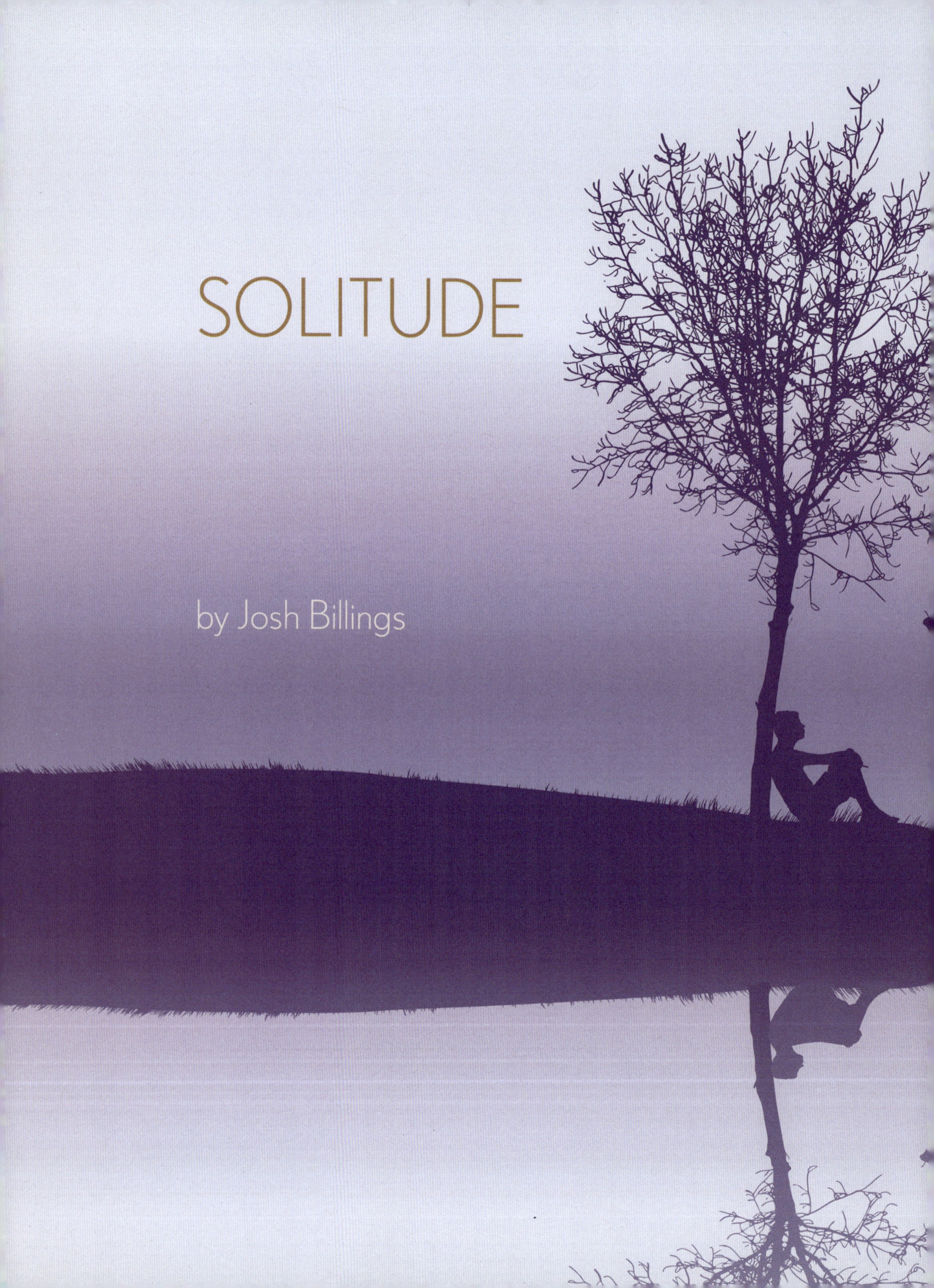
SOLITUDE
by Josh Billings

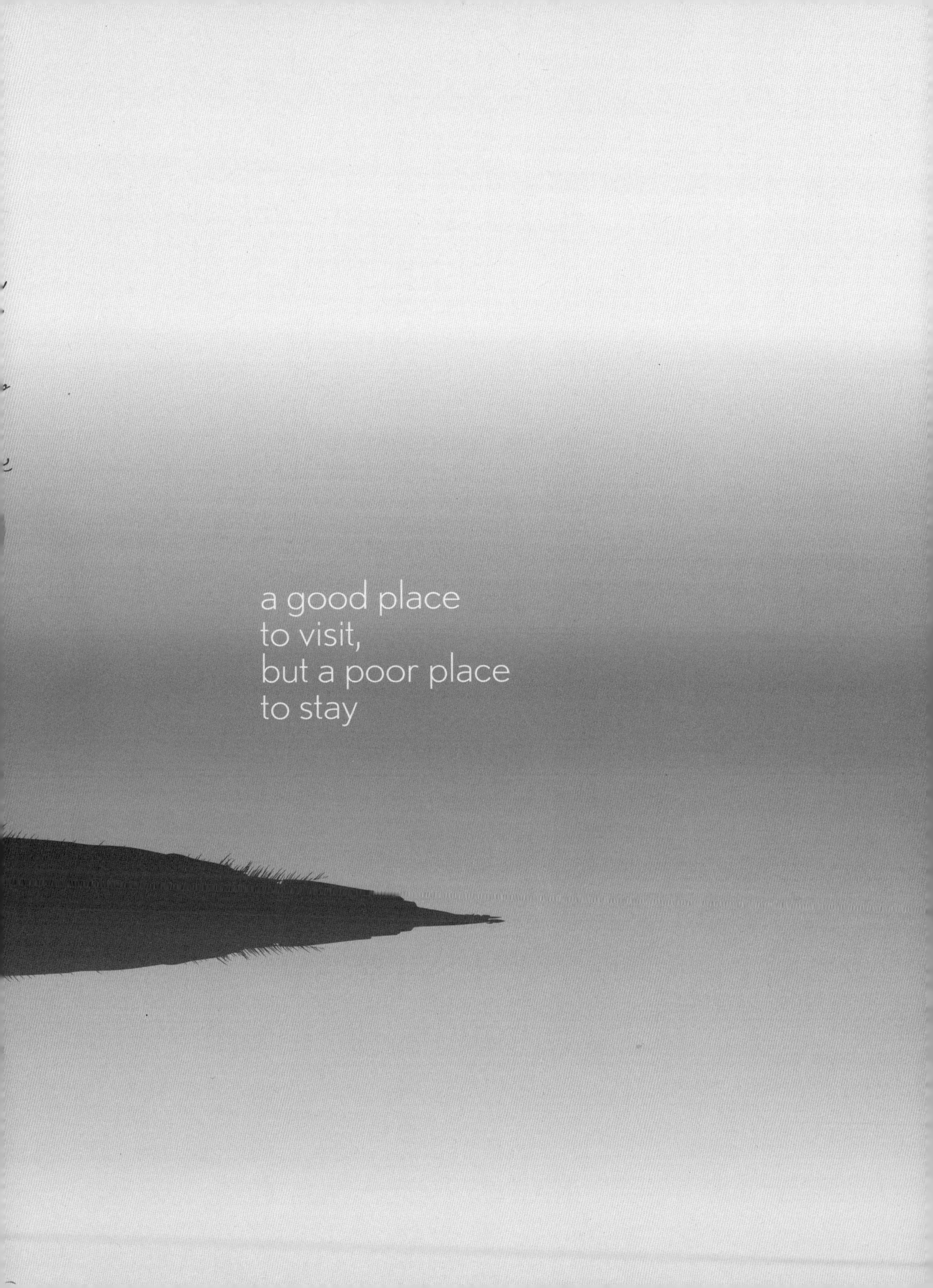

a good place
to visit,
but a poor place
to stay

SPECIAL THANKS ALSO TO:

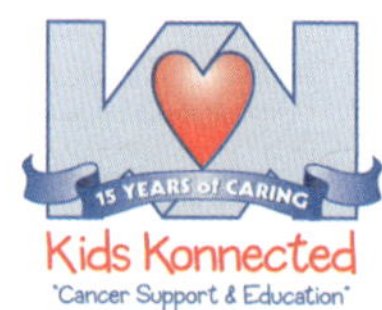

Helping kids who have a parent with cancer or lost a parent with cancer.

kidskonnected.org

- - -

Advanced Color Graphics

Brand Pixel

The C-Thru Ruler Company

dafonts.com

dictionary.com

fonts.com

K & Company

Making Memories

quotationspage.com

shutterstock.com